Fibromyalgia CFS ME MS Cancer

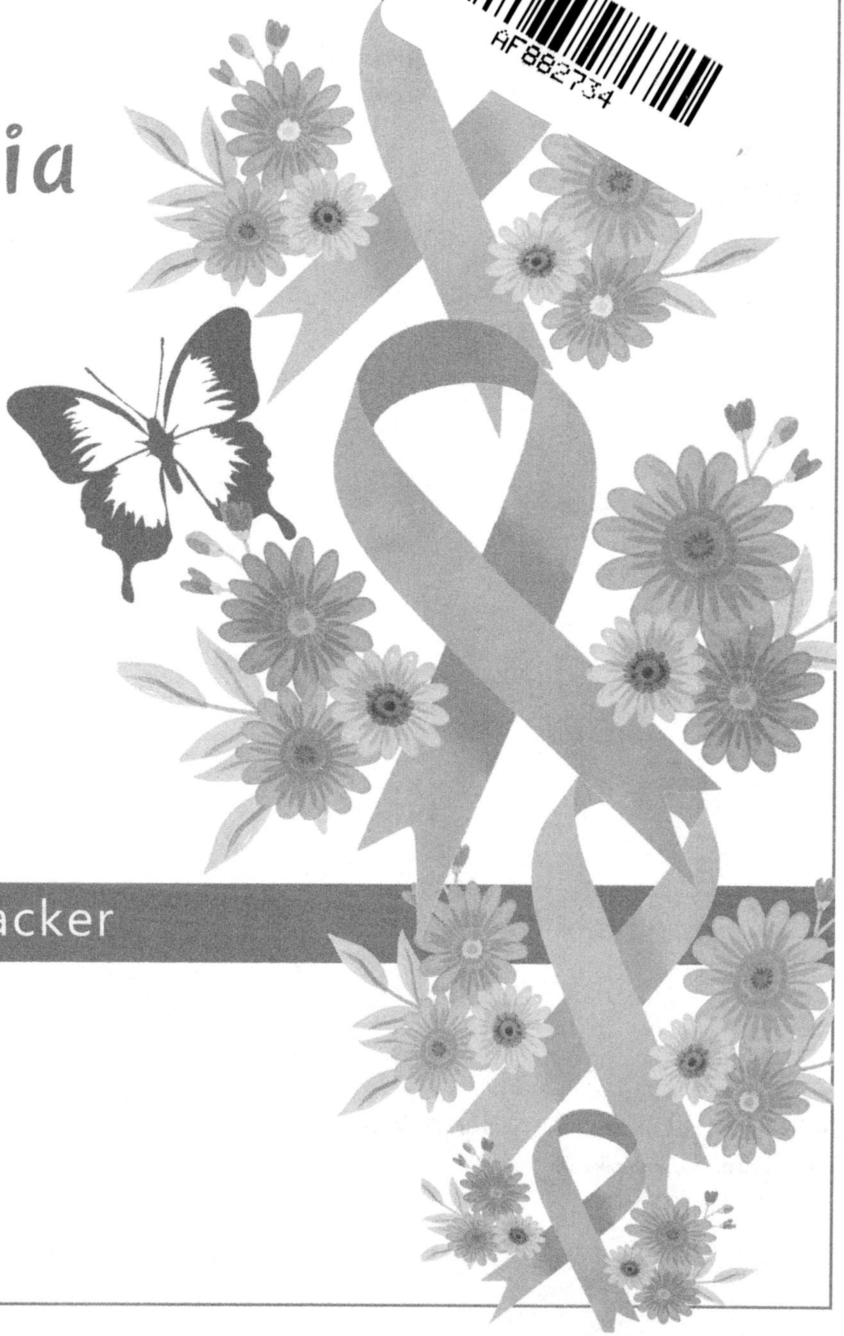

Daily Symptoms Tracker

eDiY Publishing

Fibromyalgia CFS ME MS Cancer Daily Symptoms Tracker

ISBN 13:
978-0-6486715-1-0

Images sourced, with our thanks and gratitude from:
Pixabay.com and Freepik.com

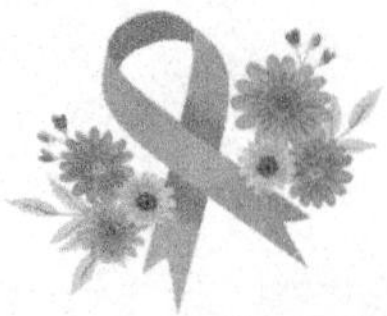

This book belongs to

....

If found, please contact

....

Personal Information

Name: ______________________________

Address: ______________________________

DOB: ______ / ______ / ______ Blood Type: ______________

Height: ______________ Weight: ______________

Medical Conditions

Allergies

Hospitalisations & Surgeries

Year

Vaccinations

Year

Emergency Contacts

Name ______________ Phone Number ______________

Relationship ______________ Alternate Number ______________

Name ______________ Phone Number ______________

Relationship ______________ Alternate Number ______________

My Medications

Medication Name: ______________________________
Treating: ______________________________
Dosage: ____________ Frequency: ____________
Date Started: ____ / ____ / ____ Date Stopped: ____ / ____ / ____
Notes ______________________________
____
____

Medication Name: ______________________________
Treating: ______________________________
Dosage: ____________ Frequency: ____________
Date Started: ____ / ____ / ____ Date Stopped: ____ / ____ / ____
Notes ______________________________
____
____

Medication Name: ______________________________
Treating: ______________________________
Dosage: ____________ Frequency: ____________
Date Started: ____ / ____ / ____ Date Stopped: ____ / ____ / ____
Notes ______________________________
____
____

My Medications

Medication Name: ______________________________

Treating: ______________________________

Dosage: ____________ Frequency: ____________

Date Started: ____ / ____ / ____ Date Stopped: ____ / ____ / ____

Notes ______________________________

____

____

Medication Name: ______________________________

Treating: ______________________________

Dosage: ____________ Frequency: ____________

Date Started: ____ / ____ / ____ Date Stopped: ____ / ____ / ____

Notes ______________________________

____

____

Medication Name: ______________________________

Treating: ______________________________

Dosage: ____________ Frequency: ____________

Date Started: ____ / ____ / ____ Date Stopped: ____ / ____ / ____

Notes ______________________________

____

____

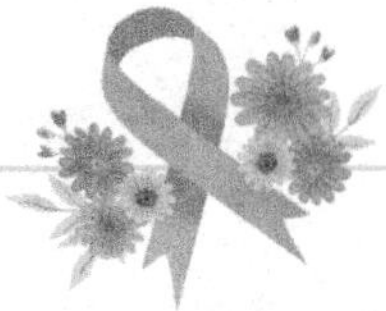

My Medications

Medication Name: ____________________
Treating: ____________________
Dosage: __________ Frequency: __________
Date Started: ____ / ____ / ____ Date Stopped: ____ / ____ / ____
Notes ____________________

Medication Name: ____________________
Treating: ____________________
Dosage: __________ Frequency: __________
Date Started: ____ / ____ / ____ Date Stopped: ____ / ____ / ____
Notes ____________________

Medication Name: ____________________
Treating: ____________________
Dosage: __________ Frequency: __________
Date Started: ____ / ____ / ____ Date Stopped: ____ / ____ / ____
Notes ____________________

My Medications

Medication Name: ______________________________
Treating: ______________________________

Dosage: ____________ Frequency: ____________
Date Started: ____ / ____ / ____ Date Stopped: ____ / ____ / ____

Notes ______________________________

____

____

Medication Name: ______________________________
Treating: ______________________________

Dosage: ____________ Frequency: ____________
Date Started: ____ / ____ / ____ Date Stopped: ____ / ____ / ____

Notes ______________________________

____

____

Medication Name: ______________________________
Treating: ______________________________

Dosage: ____________ Frequency: ____________
Date Started: ____ / ____ / ____ Date Stopped: ____ / ____ / ____

Notes ______________________________

____

____

My Medications

Medication Name: ______________________________
Treating: ______________________________

Dosage: ____________ Frequency: ____________
Date Started: ____ / ____ / ____ Date Stopped: ____ / ____ / ____

Notes ______________________________
____
____

Medication Name: ______________________________
Treating: ______________________________

Dosage: ____________ Frequency: ____________
Date Started: ____ / ____ / ____ Date Stopped: ____ / ____ / ____

Notes ______________________________
____
____

Medication Name: ______________________________
Treating: ______________________________

Dosage: ____________ Frequency: ____________
Date Started: ____ / ____ / ____ Date Stopped: ____ / ____ / ____

Notes ______________________________
____
____

Health Contacts

Name: ______________________________

Address: ______________________________

Phone Number: ______________________________

Name: ______________________________

Address: ______________________________

Phone Number: ______________________________

Name: ______________________________

Address: ______________________________

Phone Number: ______________________________

Name: ______________________________

Address: ______________________________

Phone Number: ______________________________

Name: ______________________________

Address: ______________________________

Phone Number: ______________________________

Name: ______________________________

Address: ______________________________

Phone Number: ______________________________

Name: ______________________________

Address: ______________________________

Phone Number: ______________________________

Name: ______________________________

Address: ______________________________

Phone Number: ______________________________

Appointments

With: ______________________________

Date: ______ / ______ / ______ Time: ______________

Address: ______________ Bring: ______________

Phone: ______________

With: ______________________________

Date: ______ / ______ / ______ Time: ______________

Address: ______________ Bring: ______________

Phone: ______________

With: ______________________________

Date: ______ / ______ / ______ Time: ______________

Address: ______________ Bring: ______________

Phone: ______________

With: ______________________________

Date: ______ / ______ / ______ Time: ______________

Address: ______________ Bring: ______________

Phone: ______________

Appointments

With: ____________________

Date: ______ / ______ / ______ Time: ____________________

Address: ____________________ Bring: ____________________

Phone: ____________________

With: ____________________

Date: ______ / ______ / ______ Time: ____________________

Address: ____________________ Bring: ____________________

Phone: ____________________

With: ____________________

Date: ______ / ______ / ______ Time: ____________________

Address: ____________________ Bring: ____________________

Phone: ____________________

With: ____________________

Date: ______ / ______ / ______ Time: ____________________

Address: ____________________ Bring: ____________________

Phone: ____________________

Appointments

With: ______________________________

Date: ______ / ______ / ______ Time: ______________

Address: ______________ Bring: ______________

Phone: ______________

With: ______________________________

Date: ______ / ______ / ______ Time: ______________

Address: ______________ Bring: ______________

Phone: ______________

With: ______________________________

Date: ______ / ______ / ______ Time: ______________

Address: ______________ Bring: ______________

Phone: ______________

With: ______________________________

Date: ______ / ______ / ______ Time: ______________

Address: ______________ Bring: ______________

Phone: ______________

Appointments

With: ______

Date: ____ / ____ / ____ Time: ______

Address: ______ Bring: ______

Phone: ______

With: ______

Date: ____ / ____ / ____ Time: ______

Address: ______ Bring: ______

Phone: ______

With: ______

Date: ____ / ____ / ____ Time: ______

Address: ______ Bring: ______

Phone: ______

With: ______

Date: ____ / ____ / ____ Time: ______

Address: ______ Bring: ______

Phone: ______

Appointments

With:

Date: / /

Time:

Address:

Bring:

Phone:

With:

Date: / /

Time:

Address:

Bring:

Phone:

With:

Date: / /

Time:

Address:

Bring:

Phone:

With:

Date: / /

Time:

Address:

Bring:

Phone:

Appointments

With: ____________________

Date: ____ / ____ / ____ Time: ____________

Address: ____________ Bring: ____________

Phone: ____________

With: ____________________

Date: ____ / ____ / ____ Time: ____________

Address: ____________ Bring: ____________

Phone: ____________

With: ____________________

Date: ____ / ____ / ____ Time: ____________

Address: ____________ Bring: ____________

Phone: ____________

With: ____________________

Date: ____ / ____ / ____ Time: ____________

Address: ____________ Bring: ____________

Phone: ____________

Appointments

With: ______________________________

Date: ______ / ______ / ______ Time: ______________
Address: ______________ Bring: ______________

Phone: ______________

With: ______________________________

Date: ______ / ______ / ______ Time: ______________
Address: ______________ Bring: ______________

Phone: ______________

With: ______________________________

Date: ______ / ______ / ______ Time: ______________
Address: ______________ Bring: ______________

Phone: ______________

With: ______________________________

Date: ______ / ______ / ______ Time: ______________
Address: ______________ Bring: ______________

Phone: ______________

Appointments

With: ______________________________

Date: ______ / ______ / ______ Time: ______________

Address: ______________ Bring: ______________

______________________________ ______________________________

______________________________ ______________________________

Phone: ______________________________ ______________________________

With: ______________________________

Date: ______ / ______ / ______ Time: ______________

Address: ______________ Bring: ______________

______________________________ ______________________________

______________________________ ______________________________

Phone: ______________________________ ______________________________

With: ______________________________

Date: ______ / ______ / ______ Time: ______________

Address: ______________ Bring: ______________

______________________________ ______________________________

______________________________ ______________________________

Phone: ______________________________ ______________________________

With: ______________________________

Date: ______ / ______ / ______ Time: ______________

Address: ______________ Bring: ______________

______________________________ ______________________________

______________________________ ______________________________

Phone: ______________________________ ______________________________

Daily Symptom Tracking

Daily Symptoms & Well-Being Tracker

DATE: ____ / ____ / ____

Today's Ratings

Pain	______ / 10	Anxiety	______ / 10		
Fatigue	______ / 10	Depression	______ / 10		
Weakness	______ / 10	Stress	______ / 10		
Stiffness	______ / 10	Anger	______ / 10		
General Mood	______				

Sleep

Went to bed	____ am / pm
Fell Asleep	____ am / pm
Woke up	____ am / pm
Total Hours slept	______
# of Disruptions	______

Symptoms	Relief Attempts	Results Notes

Activity

- ☐ Walk - distance ______
- ☐ Physiotherapy
- ☐ Light Exercise
- ☐ Gym
- ☐ Housework
- ☐ ______
- ☐ ______

Medications taken

- ☐ Diabetes
- ☐ Blood Pressure
- ☐ Pain Management (Prescription)
- ☐ Pain (overcounter): ______
- ☐ Natural Therapies: ______
- ☐ Other: ______
- ☐ Other: ______

Medications

- ☐ No Change
- ☐ Dosage Changed
- ☐ from ______
- ☐ to ______
- ☐ Medication Changed
  - from ______
  - to ______

DAY

Drinks & Beverages

- ☐ Milk ☐ Juice ☐ Water
- ☐ Tea ☐ Coffee ☐ Soft / Energy Drink

Hydration

Breakfast

Blood Sugar: ____
Blood Pressure: ____
Temperature: ____
Other: ____

Lunch

Blood Sugar: ____
Blood Pressure: ____
Temperature: ____
Other: ____

Dinner

Blood Sugar: ____
Blood Pressure: ____
Temperature: ____
Other: ____

Snacks

Blood Sugar: ____
Blood Pressure: ____
Temperature: ____
Other: ____

- ☐ Fruit ☐ Vegetables ☐ Ginger Tea
- ☐ Grains & Cereals ☐ Fats

Daily Symptoms & Well-Being Tracker

DATE: ____ / ____ / ____

Today's Ratings

Pain	______ / 10	Anxiety	______ / 10		
Fatigue	______ / 10	Depression	______ / 10		
Weakness	______ / 10	Stress	______ / 10		
Stiffness	______ / 10	Anger	______ / 10		
General Mood	______				

Sleep

Went to bed	____ am / pm
Fell Asleep	____ am / pm
Woke up	____ am / pm
Total Hours slept	______
# of Disruptions	______

Symptoms	Relief Attempts	Results Notes

Activity

- ☐ Walk - distance ______
- ☐ Physiotherapy
- ☐ Light Exercise
- ☐ Gym
- ☐ Housework
- ☐ ______
- ☐ ______

Medications taken

- ☐ Diabetes
- ☐ Blood Pressure
- ☐ Pain Management (Prescription)
- ☐ Pain (overcounter): ______
- ☐ Natural Therapies: ______
- ☐ Other: ______
- ☐ Other: ______

Medications

- ☐ No Change
- ☐ Dosage Changed
- ☐ from ______
- ☐ to ______
- ☐ Medication Changed
  - from ______
  - to ______

DAY

Today,'s Dietary Intake

Drinks & Beverages

- ☐ Milk ☐ Juice ☐ Water
- ☐ Tea ☐ Coffee ☐ Soft / Energy Drink

Hydration

Breakfast

Blood Sugar:
Blood Pressure:
Temperature:
Other:

Lunch

Blood Sugar:
Blood Pressure:
Temperature:
Other:

Dinner

Blood Sugar:
Blood Pressure:
Temperature:
Other:

Snacks

Blood Sugar:
Blood Pressure:
Temperature:
Other:

- ☐ Fruit ☐ Vegetables ☐ Ginger Tea
- ☐ Grains & Cereals ☐ Fats

Daily Symptoms & Well-Being Tracker

DATE: ____ / ____ / ____

Today's Ratings

Pain	______ / 10	Anxiety	______ / 10		
Fatigue	______ / 10	Depression	______ / 10		
Weakness	______ / 10	Stress	______ / 10		
Stiffness	______ / 10	Anger	______ / 10		
General Mood	______				

Sleep

Went to bed	____ am / pm
Fell Asleep	____ am / pm
Woke up	____ am / pm
Total Hours slept	______
# of Disruptions	______

Symptoms	Relief Attempts	Results Notes

Activity

- ☐ Walk - distance ______
- ☐ Physiotherapy
- ☐ Light Exercise
- ☐ Gym
- ☐ Housework
- ☐ ______
- ☐ ______

Medications taken

- ☐ Diabetes
- ☐ Blood Pressure
- ☐ Pain Management (Prescription)
- ☐ Pain (overcounter): ______
- ☐ Natural Therapies: ______
- ☐ Other: ______
- ☐ Other: ______

Medications

- ☐ No Change
- ☐ Dosage Changed
- ☐ from ______
- ☐ to ______
- ☐ Medication Changed
- from ______
- to ______

DAY

Today,'s Dietary Intake

Drinks & Beverages

- ☐ Milk ☐ Juice ☐ Water
- ☐ Tea ☐ Coffee ☐ Soft / Energy Drink

Hydration

Breakfast	Blood Sugar: ______ Blood Pressure: ______ Temperature: ______ Other: ______
Lunch	Blood Sugar: ______ Blood Pressure: ______ Temperature: ______ Other: ______
Dinner	Blood Sugar: ______ Blood Pressure: ______ Temperature: ______ Other: ______
Snacks	Blood Sugar: ______ Blood Pressure: ______ Temperature: ______ Other: ______

- ☐ Fruit ☐ Vegetables ☐ Ginger Tea
- ☐ Grains & Cereals ☐ Fats

Daily Symptoms & Well-Being Tracker

DATE: ____ / ____ / ____

Today's Ratings

Pain	______ / 10	Anxiety	______ / 10	Went to bed	____ am / pm
Fatigue	______ / 10	Depression	______ / 10	Fell Asleep	____ am / pm
Weakness	______ / 10	Stress	______ / 10	Woke up	____ am / pm
Stiffness	______ / 10	Anger	______ / 10	Total Hours slept	______
General Mood	______			# of Disruptions	______

Sleep

Symptoms	Relief Attempts	Results Notes

Activity

- ☐ Walk - distance ______
- ☐ Physiotherapy
- ☐ Light Exercise
- ☐ Gym
- ☐ Housework
- ☐ ______
- ☐ ______

Medications taken

- ☐ Diabetes
- ☐ Blood Pressure
- ☐ Pain Management (Prescription)
- ☐ Pain (overcounter): ______
- ☐ Natural Therapies: ______
- ☐ Other: ______
- ☐ Other: ______

Medications

- ☐ No Change
- ☐ Dosage Changed
- ☐ from ______
- ☐ to ______
- ☐ Medication Changed
  - from ______
  - to ______

DAY

Today,'s Dietary Intake

Drinks & Beverages

- ☐ Milk
- ☐ Juice
- ☐ Water
- ☐ Tea
- ☐ Coffee
- ☐ Soft / Energy Drink

Hydration

Breakfast

Blood Sugar: ______
Blood Pressure: ______
Temperature: ______
Other: ______

Lunch

Blood Sugar: ______
Blood Pressure: ______
Temperature: ______
Other: ______

Dinner

Blood Sugar: ______
Blood Pressure: ______
Temperature: ______
Other: ______

Snacks

Blood Sugar: ______
Blood Pressure: ______
Temperature: ______
Other: ______

- ☐ Fruit
- ☐ Vegetables
- ☐ Ginger Tea
- ☐ Grains & Cereals
- ☐ Fats

Daily Symptoms & Well-Being Tracker

DATE: ____ / ____ / ____

Today's Ratings

Pain ________ / 10

Fatigue ________ / 10

Weakness ________ / 10

Stiffness ________ / 10

General Mood ____________

Anxiety ________ / 10

Depression ________ / 10

Stress ________ / 10

Anger ________ / 10

Sleep

Went to bed ____ am / pm

Fell Asleep ____ am / pm

Woke up ____ am / pm

Total Hours slept ____________

# of Disruptions ____________

Symptoms	Relief Attempts	Results Notes

Activity

- ☐ Walk - distance ________
- ☐ Physiotherapy
- ☐ Light Exercise
- ☐ Gym
- ☐ Housework
- ☐ ____________
- ☐ ____________

Medications taken

- ☐ Diabetes
- ☐ Blood Pressure
- ☐ Pain Management (Prescription)
- ☐ Pain (overcounter): ____________
- ☐ Natural Therapies: ____________
- ☐ Other: ____________
- ☐ Other: ____________

Medications

- ☐ No Change
- ☐ Dosage Changed
- ☐ from ____________
- ☐ to ____________
- ☐ Medication Changed
  - from ____________
  - to ____________

DAY

Today,'s Dietary Intake

Drinks & Beverages

- ☐ Milk ☐ Juice ☐ Water
- ☐ Tea ☐ Coffee ☐ Soft / Energy Drink

Hydration

Breakfast

Blood Sugar: ______

Blood Pressure: ______

Temperature: ______

Other: ______

Lunch

Blood Sugar: ______

Blood Pressure: ______

Temperature: ______

Other: ______

Dinner

Blood Sugar: ______

Blood Pressure: ______

Temperature: ______

Other: ______

Snacks

Blood Sugar: ______

Blood Pressure: ______

Temperature: ______

Other: ______

- ☐ Fruit ☐ Vegetables ☐ Ginger Tea
- ☐ Grains & Cereals ☐ Fats

Daily Symptoms & Well-Being Tracker

DATE: ____ / ____ / ____

Today's Ratings

Pain	____ / 10	Anxiety	____ / 10	Went to bed	____ am / pm
Fatigue	____ / 10	Depression	____ / 10	Fell Asleep	____ am / pm
Weakness	____ / 10	Stress	____ / 10	Woke up	____ am / pm
Stiffness	____ / 10	Anger	____ / 10	Total Hours slept	____
General Mood	____			# of Disruptions	____

Sleep

Symptoms	Relief Attempts	Results Notes

Activity

- ☐ Walk - distance ____
- ☐ Physiotherapy
- ☐ Light Exercise
- ☐ Gym
- ☐ Housework
- ☐ ____
- ☐ ____

Medications taken

- ☐ Diabetes
- ☐ Blood Pressure
- ☐ Pain Management (Prescription)
- ☐ Pain (overcounter): ____
- ☐ Natural Therapies: ____
- ☐ Other: ____
- ☐ Other: ____

Medications

- ☐ No Change
- ☐ Dosage Changed
- ☐ from ____
- ☐ to ____
- ☐ Medication Changed
- from ____
- to ____

DAY

Today,'s Dietary Intake

Drinks & Beverages

- ☐ Milk ☐ Juice ☐ Water
- ☐ Tea ☐ Coffee ☐ Soft / Energy Drink

Hydration

Breakfast	
	Blood Sugar: ______
	Blood Pressure: ______
	Temperature: ______
	Other: ______

Lunch	
	Blood Sugar: ______
	Blood Pressure: ______
	Temperature: ______
	Other: ______

Dinner	
	Blood Sugar: ______
	Blood Pressure: ______
	Temperature: ______
	Other: ______

Snacks	
	Blood Sugar: ______
	Blood Pressure: ______
	Temperature: ______
	Other: ______

- ☐ Fruit ☐ Vegetables ☐ Ginger Tea
- ☐ Grains & Cereals ☐ Fats

Daily Symptoms & Well-Being Tracker

DATE: ____ / ____ / ____

Today's Ratings

Pain	______ / 10	Anxiety	______ / 10
Fatigue	______ / 10	Depression	______ / 10
Weakness	______ / 10	Stress	______ / 10
Stiffness	______ / 10	Anger	______ / 10
General Mood	______		

Sleep

Went to bed	____ am / pm
Fell Asleep	____ am / pm
Woke up	____ am / pm
Total Hours slept	______
# of Disruptions	______

Symptoms	Relief Attempts	Results Notes

Activity

- ☐ Walk - distance ______
- ☐ Physiotherapy
- ☐ Light Exercise
- ☐ Gym
- ☐ Housework
- ☐ ______
- ☐ ______

Medications taken

- ☐ Diabetes
- ☐ Blood Pressure
- ☐ Pain Management (Prescription)
- ☐ Pain (overcounter): ______
- ☐ Natural Therapies: ______
- ☐ Other: ______
- ☐ Other: ______

Medications

- ☐ No Change
- ☐ Dosage Changed
- ☐ from ______
- ☐ to ______
- ☐ Medication Changed
  - from ______
  - to ______

DAY

Today,'s Dietary Intake

Drinks & Beverages

- ☐ Milk ☐ Juice ☐ Water
- ☐ Tea ☐ Coffee ☐ Soft / Energy Drink

Hydration

Breakfast

Blood Sugar: ______
Blood Pressure: ______
Temperature: ______
Other: ______

Lunch

Blood Sugar: ______
Blood Pressure: ______
Temperature: ______
Other: ______

Dinner

Blood Sugar: ______
Blood Pressure: ______
Temperature: ______
Other: ______

Snacks

Blood Sugar: ______
Blood Pressure: ______
Temperature: ______
Other: ______

- ☐ Fruit ☐ Vegetables ☐ Ginger Tea
- ☐ Grains & Cereals ☐ Fats

Weekly Summary

	Monday	Tuesday	Wednesday	Thursday	Friday	Saturday	Sunday
Pain							
Fatigue							
Weakness							
Stiffness							
Sleep (total Hours)							
# Disruptions							

Instructions:

Use the dots and dashes below to graph your ratings for the week – it helps to see things visually.

The bottom -- equals 0; the middle -- equals 5; and the top ◆ equals 10

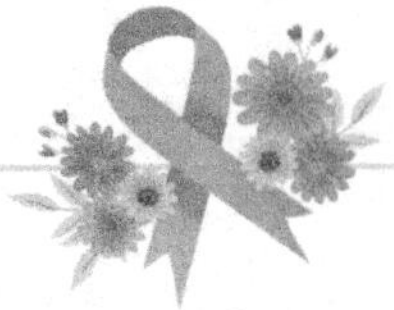

Weekly Summary

	Monday	Tuesday	Wednesday	Thursday	Friday	Saturday	Sunday
Anxiety							
Depression							
Stress							
Anger							
Brain Fog / Forgetfulness							

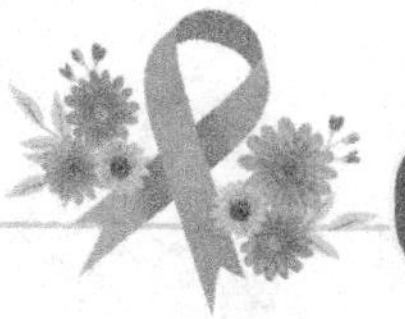

Daily Symptoms & Well-Being Tracker

DATE: ____ / ____ / ____

Today's Ratings

Pain	______ / 10	Anxiety	______ / 10
Fatigue	______ / 10	Depression	______ / 10
Weakness	______ / 10	Stress	______ / 10
Stiffness	______ / 10	Anger	______ / 10
General Mood	______		

Sleep

Went to bed	____ am / pm
Fell Asleep	____ am / pm
Woke up	____ am / pm
Total Hours slept	______
# of Disruptions	______

Symptoms	Relief Attempts	Results Notes

Activity

- ☐ Walk - distance ______
- ☐ Physiotherapy
- ☐ Light Exercise
- ☐ Gym
- ☐ Housework
- ☐ ______
- ☐ ______

Medications taken

- ☐ Diabetes
- ☐ Blood Pressure
- ☐ Pain Management (Prescription)
- ☐ Pain (overcounter): ______
- ☐ Natural Therapies: ______
- ☐ Other: ______
- ☐ Other: ______

Medications

- ☐ No Change
- ☐ Dosage Changed
- ☐ from ______
- ☐ to ______
- ☐ Medication Changed
  - from ______
  - to ______

DAY

Today,'s Dietary Intake

Drinks & Beverages

☐ Milk ☐ Juice ☐ Water

☐ Tea ☐ Coffee ☐ Soft / Energy Drink

Hydration

Breakfast

Blood Sugar: ____________

Blood Pressure: ____________

Temperature: ____________

Other: ____________

Lunch

Blood Sugar: ____________

Blood Pressure: ____________

Temperature: ____________

Other: ____________

Dinner

Blood Sugar: ____________

Blood Pressure: ____________

Temperature: ____________

Other: ____________

Snacks

Blood Sugar: ____________

Blood Pressure: ____________

Temperature: ____________

Other: ____________

☐ Fruit ☐ Vegetables ☐ Ginger Tea

☐ Grains & Cereals ☐ Fats

Daily Symptoms & Well-Being Tracker

DATE: ____ / ____ / ____

Today's Ratings

Pain	______ / 10	Anxiety	______ / 10		
Fatigue	______ / 10	Depression	______ / 10		
Weakness	______ / 10	Stress	______ / 10		
Stiffness	______ / 10	Anger	______ / 10		
General Mood	______				

Sleep

Went to bed ______ am / pm

Fell Asleep ______ am / pm

Woke up ______ am / pm

Total Hours slept ______

# of Disruptions ______

Symptoms	Relief Attempts	Results Notes

Activity

- ☐ Walk - distance ______
- ☐ Physiotherapy
- ☐ Light Exercise
- ☐ Gym
- ☐ Housework
- ☐ ______
- ☐ ______

Medications taken

- ☐ Diabetes
- ☐ Blood Pressure
- ☐ Pain Management (Prescription)
- ☐ Pain (overcounter): ______
- ☐ Natural Therapies: ______
- ☐ Other: ______
- ☐ Other: ______

Medications

- ☐ No Change
- ☐ Dosage Changed
- ☐ from ______
- ☐ to ______
- ☐ Medication Changed
- from ______
- to ______

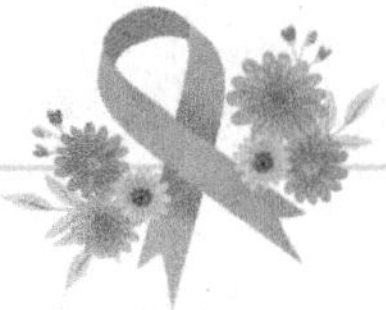

DAY

Today.'s Dietary Intake

Drinks & Beverages

- ☐ Milk ☐ Juice ☐ Water
- ☐ Tea ☐ Coffee ☐ Soft / Energy Drink

Hydration

Breakfast

Blood Sugar: ______
Blood Pressure: ______
Temperature: ______
Other: ______

Lunch

Blood Sugar: ______
Blood Pressure: ______
Temperature: ______
Other: ______

Dinner

Blood Sugar: ______
Blood Pressure: ______
Temperature: ______
Other: ______

Snacks

Blood Sugar: ______
Blood Pressure: ______
Temperature: ______
Other: ______

- ☐ Fruit ☐ Vegetables ☐ Ginger Tea
- ☐ Grains & Cereals ☐ Fats

Daily Symptoms & Well-Being Tracker

DATE: ____ / ____ / ____

Today's Ratings

Pain	____ / 10	Anxiety	____ / 10		
Fatigue	____ / 10	Depression	____ / 10		
Weakness	____ / 10	Stress	____ / 10		
Stiffness	____ / 10	Anger	____ / 10		
General Mood	____				

Sleep

Went to bed	____ am / pm
Fell Asleep	____ am / pm
Woke up	____ am / pm
Total Hours slept	____
# of Disruptions	____

Symptoms	Relief Attempts	Results Notes

Activity

- ☐ Walk - distance ____
- ☐ Physiotherapy
- ☐ Light Exercise
- ☐ Gym
- ☐ Housework
- ☐ ____
- ☐ ____

Medications taken

- ☐ Diabetes
- ☐ Blood Pressure
- ☐ Pain Management (Prescription)
- ☐ Pain (overcounter): ____
- ☐ Natural Therapies: ____
- ☐ Other: ____
- ☐ Other: ____

Medications

- ☐ No Change
- ☐ Dosage Changed
- ☐ from ____
- ☐ to ____
- ☐ Medication Changed
- from ____
- to ____

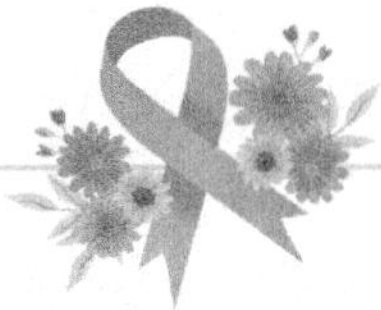

DAY

Today,'s Dietary Intake

Drinks & Beverages

- ☐ Milk ☐ Juice ☐ Water
- ☐ Tea ☐ Coffee ☐ Soft / Energy Drink

Hydration

Breakfast

Blood Sugar: ____________
Blood Pressure: ____________
Temperature: ____________
Other: ____________

Lunch

Blood Sugar: ____________
Blood Pressure: ____________
Temperature: ____________
Other: ____________

Dinner

Blood Sugar: ____________
Blood Pressure: ____________
Temperature: ____________
Other: ____________

Snacks

Blood Sugar: ____________
Blood Pressure: ____________
Temperature: ____________
Other: ____________

- ☐ Fruit ☐ Vegetables ☐ Ginger Tea
- ☐ Grains & Cereals ☐ Fats

Daily Symptoms & Well-Being Tracker

DATE: ____ / ____ / ____

Today's Ratings

Pain	______ / 10	Anxiety	______ / 10	Went to bed	____ am / pm
Fatigue	______ / 10	Depression	______ / 10	Fell Asleep	____ am / pm
Weakness	______ / 10	Stress	______ / 10	Woke up	____ am / pm
Stiffness	______ / 10	Anger	______ / 10	Total Hours slept	______
General Mood	______			# of Disruptions	______

Sleep

Symptoms	Relief Attempts	Results Notes

Activity

- ☐ Walk - distance ______
- ☐ Physiotherapy
- ☐ Light Exercise
- ☐ Gym
- ☐ Housework
- ☐ ______
- ☐ ______

Medications taken

- ☐ Diabetes
- ☐ Blood Pressure
- ☐ Pain Management (Prescription)
- ☐ Pain (overcounter): ______
- ☐ Natural Therapies: ______
- ☐ Other: ______
- ☐ Other: ______

Medications

- ☐ No Change
- ☐ Dosage Changed
- ☐ from ______
- ☐ to ______
- ☐ Medication Changed
  - from ______
  - to ______

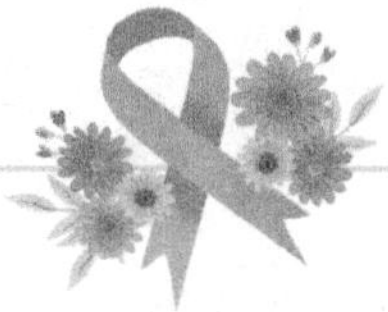

Daily Symptoms Tracker

Today,'s Dietary Intake

DAY

Drinks & Beverages

- ☐ Milk ☐ Juice ☐ Water
- ☐ Tea ☐ Coffee ☐ Soft / Energy Drink

Hydration

Breakfast

Blood Sugar: ______
Blood Pressure: ______
Temperature: ______
Other: ______

Lunch

Blood Sugar: ______
Blood Pressure: ______
Temperature: ______
Other: ______

Dinner

Blood Sugar: ______
Blood Pressure: ______
Temperature: ______
Other: ______

Snacks

Blood Sugar: ______
Blood Pressure: ______
Temperature: ______
Other: ______

- ☐ Fruit ☐ Vegetables ☐ Ginger Tea
- ☐ Grains & Cereals ☐ Fats

Daily Symptoms & Well-Being Tracker

DATE: ____ / ____ / ____

Today's Ratings

Pain ________ / 10
Fatigue ________ / 10
Weakness ________ / 10
Stiffness ________ / 10
General Mood ____________

Anxiety ________ / 10
Depression ________ / 10
Stress ________ / 10
Anger ________ / 10

Sleep

Went to bed _____ am / pm
Fell Asleep _____ am / pm
Woke up _____ am / pm
Total Hours slept ____________
# of Disruptions ____________

Symptoms	Relief Attempts	Results Notes

Activity

- ☐ Walk - distance ________
- ☐ Physiotherapy
- ☐ Light Exercise
- ☐ Gym
- ☐ Housework
- ☐ ____________
- ☐ ____________

Medications taken

- ☐ Diabetes
- ☐ Blood Pressure
- ☐ Pain Management (Prescription)
- ☐ Pain (overcounter): ____________
- ☐ Natural Therapies: ____________
- ☐ Other: ____________
- ☐ Other: ____________

Medications

- ☐ No Change
- ☐ Dosage Changed
- ☐ from ____________
- ☐ to ____________
- ☐ Medication Changed

from ____________

to ____________

Today,'s Dietary Intake

DAY

Drinks & Beverages

- ☐ Milk ☐ Juice ☐ Water
- ☐ Tea ☐ Coffee ☐ Soft / Energy Drink

Hydration

☐ ☐ ☐ ☐ ☐ ☐ ☐

Meal	Readings
Breakfast	Blood Sugar: ______ Blood Pressure: ______ Temperature: ______ Other: ______
Lunch	Blood Sugar: ______ Blood Pressure: ______ Temperature: ______ Other: ______
Dinner	Blood Sugar: ______ Blood Pressure: ______ Temperature: ______ Other: ______
Snacks	Blood Sugar: ______ Blood Pressure: ______ Temperature: ______ Other: ______

- ☐ Fruit ☐ Vegetables ☐ Ginger Tea
- ☐ Grains & Cereals ☐ Fats

Daily Symptoms & Well-Being Tracker

DATE: ____ / ____ / ____

Today's Ratings

Pain	______ / 10	Anxiety	______ / 10	Went to bed	____ am / pm
Fatigue	______ / 10	Depression	______ / 10	Fell Asleep	____ am / pm
Weakness	______ / 10	Stress	______ / 10	Woke up	____ am / pm
Stiffness	______ / 10	Anger	______ / 10	Total Hours slept	______
General Mood	______			# of Disruptions	______

Symptoms	Relief Attempts	Results Notes

Activity

- ☐ Walk - distance ______
- ☐ Physiotherapy
- ☐ Light Exercise
- ☐ Gym
- ☐ Housework
- ☐ ______
- ☐ ______

Medications taken

- ☐ Diabetes
- ☐ Blood Pressure
- ☐ Pain Management (Prescription)
- ☐ Pain (overcounter): ______
- ☐ Natural Therapies: ______
- ☐ Other: ______
- ☐ Other: ______

Medications

- ☐ No Change
- ☐ Dosage Changed
- ☐ from ______
- ☐ to ______
- ☐ Medication Changed
  - from ______
  - to ______

DAY

Today,'s Dietary Intake

Drinks & Beverages

- ☐ Milk
- ☐ Juice
- ☐ Water
- ☐ Tea
- ☐ Coffee
- ☐ Soft / Energy Drink

Hydration

Breakfast

Blood Sugar: ______

Blood Pressure: ______

Temperature: ______

Other: ______

Lunch

Blood Sugar: ______

Blood Pressure: ______

Temperature: ______

Other: ______

Dinner

Blood Sugar: ______

Blood Pressure: ______

Temperature: ______

Other: ______

Snacks

Blood Sugar: ______

Blood Pressure: ______

Temperature: ______

Other: ______

- ☐ Fruit
- ☐ Vegetables
- ☐ Ginger Tea
- ☐ Grains & Cereals
- ☐ Fats

Daily Symptoms & Well-Being Tracker

DATE: ____ / ____ / ____

Today's Ratings

Pain	______ / 10	Anxiety	______ / 10
Fatigue	______ / 10	Depression	______ / 10
Weakness	______ / 10	Stress	______ / 10
Stiffness	______ / 10	Anger	______ / 10
General Mood	______		

Sleep

Went to bed	____ am / pm
Fell Asleep	____ am / pm
Woke up	____ am / pm
Total Hours slept	______
# of Disruptions	______

Symptoms	Relief Attempts	Results Notes

Activity

- ☐ Walk - distance ______
- ☐ Physiotherapy
- ☐ Light Exercise
- ☐ Gym
- ☐ Housework
- ☐ ______
- ☐ ______

Medications taken

- ☐ Diabetes
- ☐ Blood Pressure
- ☐ Pain Management (Prescription)
- ☐ Pain (overcounter): ______
- ☐ Natural Therapies: ______
- ☐ Other: ______
- ☐ Other: ______

Medications

- ☐ No Change
- ☐ Dosage Changed
- ☐ from ______
- ☐ to ______
- ☐ Medication Changed
  - from ______
  - to ______

Today,'s Dietary Intake

DAY

Drinks & Beverages

- ☐ Milk ☐ Juice ☐ Water
- ☐ Tea ☐ Coffee ☐ Soft / Energy Drink

Hydration

Breakfast

Blood Sugar: ______
Blood Pressure: ______
Temperature: ______
Other: ______

Lunch

Blood Sugar: ______
Blood Pressure: ______
Temperature: ______
Other: ______

Dinner

Blood Sugar: ______
Blood Pressure: ______
Temperature: ______
Other: ______

Snacks

Blood Sugar: ______
Blood Pressure: ______
Temperature: ______
Other: ______

- ☐ Fruit ☐ Vegetables ☐ Ginger Tea
- ☐ Grains & Cereals ☐ Fats

Weekly Summary

	Monday	Tuesday	Wednesday	Thursday	Friday	Saturday	Sunday
Pain							
Fatigue							
Weakness							
Stiffness							
Sleep (total Hours)							
# Disruptions							

Instructions:

Use the dots and dashes below to graph your ratings for the week – it helps to see things visually.

The bottom -- equals 0; the middle -- equals 5; and the top ◆ equals 10

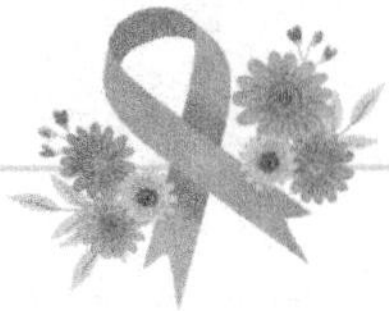

Weekly Summary

	Monday	Tuesday	Wednesday	Thursday	Friday	Saturday	Sunday
Anxiety							
Depression							
Stress							
Anger							
Brain Fog / Forgetfulness							

Daily Symptoms & Well-Being Tracker

DATE: ____ / ____ / ____

Today's Ratings

Pain	______ / 10	Anxiety	______ / 10
Fatigue	______ / 10	Depression	______ / 10
Weakness	______ / 10	Stress	______ / 10
Stiffness	______ / 10	Anger	______ / 10
General Mood	______		

Sleep

Went to bed	____ am / pm
Fell Asleep	____ am / pm
Woke up	____ am / pm
Total Hours slept	______
# of Disruptions	______

Symptoms	Relief Attempts	Results Notes

Activity

- ☐ Walk - distance ______
- ☐ Physiotherapy
- ☐ Light Exercise
- ☐ Gym
- ☐ Housework
- ☐ ______
- ☐ ______

Medications taken

- ☐ Diabetes
- ☐ Blood Pressure
- ☐ Pain Management (Prescription)
- ☐ Pain (overcounter): ______
- ☐ Natural Therapies: ______
- ☐ Other: ______
- ☐ Other: ______

Medications

- ☐ No Change
- ☐ Dosage Changed
- ☐ from ______
- ☐ to ______
- ☐ Medication Changed
  - from ______
  - to ______

Today,'s Dietary Intake

DAY

Drinks & Beverages

- ☐ Milk
- ☐ Juice
- ☐ Water
- ☐ Tea
- ☐ Coffee
- ☐ Soft / Energy Drink

Hydration

Breakfast

Blood Sugar: ______
Blood Pressure: ______
Temperature: ______
Other: ______

Lunch

Blood Sugar: ______
Blood Pressure: ______
Temperature: ______
Other: ______

Dinner

Blood Sugar: ______
Blood Pressure: ______
Temperature: ______
Other: ______

Snacks

Blood Sugar: ______
Blood Pressure: ______
Temperature: ______
Other: ______

- ☐ Fruit
- ☐ Vegetables
- ☐ Ginger Tea
- ☐ Grains & Cereals
- ☐ Fats

Daily Symptoms & Well-Being Tracker

DATE: ____ / ____ / ____

Today's Ratings

Pain ________ / 10
Fatigue ________ / 10
Weakness ________ / 10
Stiffness ________ / 10
General Mood ____________

Anxiety ________ / 10
Depression ________ / 10
Stress ________ / 10
Anger ________ / 10

Sleep

Went to bed _____ am / pm
Fell Asleep _____ am / pm
Woke up _____ am / pm
Total Hours slept ____________
# of Disruptions ____________

Symptoms	Relief Attempts	Results Notes

Activity

- ☐ Walk - distance ________
- ☐ Physiotherapy
- ☐ Light Exercise
- ☐ Gym
- ☐ Housework
- ☐ ____________
- ☐ ____________

Medications taken

- ☐ Diabetes
- ☐ Blood Pressure
- ☐ Pain Management (Prescription)
- ☐ Pain (overcounter): ____________
- ☐ Natural Therapies: ____________
- ☐ Other: ____________
- ☐ Other: ____________

Medications

- ☐ No Change
- ☐ Dosage Changed
- ☐ from ____________
- ☐ to ____________
- ☐ Medication Changed
  - from ____________
  - to ____________

DAY

Drinks & Beverages

- ☐ Milk ☐ Juice ☐ Water
- ☐ Tea ☐ Coffee ☐ Soft / Energy Drink

Hydration

Breakfast

Blood Sugar: ____________

Blood Pressure: ____________

Temperature: ____________

Other: ____________

Lunch

Blood Sugar: ____________

Blood Pressure: ____________

Temperature: ____________

Other: ____________

Dinner

Blood Sugar: ____________

Blood Pressure: ____________

Temperature: ____________

Other: ____________

Snacks

Blood Sugar: ____________

Blood Pressure: ____________

Temperature: ____________

Other: ____________

- ☐ Fruit ☐ Vegetables ☐ Ginger Tea
- ☐ Grains & Cereals ☐ Fats

Daily Symptoms & Well-Being Tracker

DATE: ____ / ____ / ____

Today's Ratings

Pain	______ / 10	Anxiety	______ / 10	Went to bed	____ am / pm
Fatigue	______ / 10	Depression	______ / 10	Fell Asleep	____ am / pm
Weakness	______ / 10	Stress	______ / 10	Woke up	____ am / pm
Stiffness	______ / 10	Anger	______ / 10	Total Hours slept	______
General Mood	______			# of Disruptions	______

Symptoms	Relief Attempts	Results Notes

Activity	Medications taken	Medications
☐ Walk - distance ______	☐ Diabetes	☐ No Change
☐ Physiotherapy	☐ Blood Pressure	☐ Dosage Changed
☐ Light Exercise	☐ Pain Management (Prescription)	☐ from ______
☐ Gym	☐ Pain (overcounter): ______	☐ to ______
☐ Housework	☐ Natural Therapies: ______	☐ Medication Changed
☐ ______	☐ Other: ______	from ______
☐ ______	☐ Other: ______	to ______

DAY

Today,'s Dietary Intake

Drinks & Beverages

- ☐ Milk ☐ Juice ☐ Water
- ☐ Tea ☐ Coffee ☐ Soft / Energy Drink

Hydration

Breakfast

Blood Sugar: ____________

Blood Pressure: ____________

Temperature: ____________

Other: ____________

Lunch

Blood Sugar: ____________

Blood Pressure: ____________

Temperature: ____________

Other: ____________

Dinner

Blood Sugar: ____________

Blood Pressure: ____________

Temperature: ____________

Other: ____________

Snacks

Blood Sugar: ____________

Blood Pressure: ____________

Temperature: ____________

Other: ____________

- ☐ Fruit ☐ Vegetables ☐ Ginger Tea
- ☐ Grains & Cereals ☐ Fats

Daily Symptoms & Well-Being Tracker

DATE: ____ / ____ / ____

Today's Ratings

Pain ________ / 10
Fatigue ________ / 10
Weakness ________ / 10
Stiffness ________ / 10
General Mood ________

Anxiety ________ / 10
Depression ________ / 10
Stress ________ / 10
Anger ________ / 10

Sleep

Went to bed ____ am / pm
Fell Asleep ____ am / pm
Woke up ____ am / pm
Total Hours slept ________
# of Disruptions ________

Symptoms	Relief Attempts	Results Notes

Activity

- ☐ Walk - distance ________
- ☐ Physiotherapy
- ☐ Light Exercise
- ☐ Gym
- ☐ Housework
- ☐ ________
- ☐ ________

Medications taken

- ☐ Diabetes
- ☐ Blood Pressure
- ☐ Pain Management (Prescription)
- ☐ Pain (overcounter): ________
- ☐ Natural Therapies: ________
- ☐ Other: ________
- ☐ Other: ________

Medications

- ☐ No Change
- ☐ Dosage Changed
- ☐ from ________
- ☐ to ________
- ☐ Medication Changed

  from ________

  to ________

DAY

Today,'s Dietary Intake

Drinks & Beverages

- ☐ Milk ☐ Juice ☐ Water
- ☐ Tea ☐ Coffee ☐ Soft / Energy Drink

Hydration

☐ ☐ ☐ ☐ ☐ ☐ ☐

Breakfast

	Blood Sugar: ______
______	Blood Pressure: ______
______	Temperature: ______
______	Other: ______

Lunch

______	Blood Sugar: ______
______	Blood Pressure: ______
______	Temperature: ______
______	Other: ______

Dinner

______	Blood Sugar: ______
______	Blood Pressure: ______
______	Temperature: ______
______	Other: ______
______	

Snacks

______	Blood Sugar: ______
______	Blood Pressure: ______
______	Temperature: ______
______	Other: ______

- ☐ Fruit ☐ Vegetables ☐ Ginger Tea
- ☐ Grains & Cereals ☐ Fats

Daily Symptoms & Well-Being Tracker

DATE: ____ / ____ / ____

Today's Ratings

Pain	____ / 10	Anxiety	____ / 10	Went to bed	____ am / pm
Fatigue	____ / 10	Depression	____ / 10	Fell Asleep	____ am / pm
Weakness	____ / 10	Stress	____ / 10	Woke up	____ am / pm
Stiffness	____ / 10	Anger	____ / 10	Total Hours slept	____
General Mood	____			# of Disruptions	____

Symptoms	Relief Attempts	Results Notes

Activity

- ☐ Walk - distance ____
- ☐ Physiotherapy
- ☐ Light Exercise
- ☐ Gym
- ☐ Housework
- ☐ ____
- ☐ ____

Medications taken

- ☐ Diabetes
- ☐ Blood Pressure
- ☐ Pain Management (Prescription)
- ☐ Pain (overcounter): ____
- ☐ Natural Therapies: ____
- ☐ Other: ____
- ☐ Other: ____

Medications

- ☐ No Change
- ☐ Dosage Changed
- ☐ from ____
- ☐ to ____
- ☐ Medication Changed
  - from ____
  - to ____

Today,'s Dietary Intake

DAY

Drinks & Beverages

- ☐ Milk
- ☐ Juice
- ☐ Water
- ☐ Tea
- ☐ Coffee
- ☐ Soft / Energy Drink

Hydration

Breakfast

Blood Sugar: ____________

Blood Pressure: ____________

Temperature: ____________

Other: ____________

Lunch

Blood Sugar: ____________

Blood Pressure: ____________

Temperature: ____________

Other: ____________

Dinner

Blood Sugar: ____________

Blood Pressure: ____________

Temperature: ____________

Other: ____________

Snacks

Blood Sugar: ____________

Blood Pressure: ____________

Temperature: ____________

Other: ____________

- ☐ Fruit
- ☐ Vegetables
- ☐ Ginger Tea
- ☐ Grains & Cereals
- ☐ Fats

Daily Symptoms & Well-Being Tracker

DATE: ____ / ____ / ____

Today's Ratings

Pain	____ / 10	Anxiety	____ / 10	
Fatigue	____ / 10	Depression	____ / 10	
Weakness	____ / 10	Stress	____ / 10	
Stiffness	____ / 10	Anger	____ / 10	
General Mood	____			

Sleep

Went to bed	____ am / pm
Fell Asleep	____ am / pm
Woke up	____ am / pm
Total Hours slept	____
# of Disruptions	____

Symptoms	Relief Attempts	Results Notes

Activity

- ☐ Walk - distance ____
- ☐ Physiotherapy
- ☐ Light Exercise
- ☐ Gym
- ☐ Housework
- ☐ ____
- ☐ ____

Medications taken

- ☐ Diabetes
- ☐ Blood Pressure
- ☐ Pain Management (Prescription)
- ☐ Pain (overcounter): ____
- ☐ Natural Therapies: ____
- ☐ Other: ____
- ☐ Other: ____

Medications

- ☐ No Change
- ☐ Dosage Changed
- ☐ from ____
- ☐ to ____
- ☐ Medication Changed
  - from ____
  - to ____

Today,'s Dietary Intake

DAY

Drinks & Beverages

- ☐ Milk ☐ Juice ☐ Water
- ☐ Tea ☐ Coffee ☐ Soft / Energy Drink

Hydration

Breakfast

Blood Sugar: ____________
Blood Pressure: ____________
Temperature: ____________
Other: ____________

Lunch

Blood Sugar: ____________
Blood Pressure: ____________
Temperature: ____________
Other: ____________

Dinner

Blood Sugar: ____________
Blood Pressure: ____________
Temperature: ____________
Other: ____________

Snacks

Blood Sugar: ____________
Blood Pressure: ____________
Temperature: ____________
Other: ____________

- ☐ Fruit ☐ Vegetables ☐ Ginger Tea
- ☐ Grains & Cereals ☐ Fats

Daily Symptoms & Well-Being Tracker

DATE: ____ / ____ / ____

Today's Ratings

Pain	______ / 10	Anxiety	______ / 10		
Fatigue	______ / 10	Depression	______ / 10		
Weakness	______ / 10	Stress	______ / 10		
Stiffness	______ / 10	Anger	______ / 10		
General Mood	______				

Sleep

Went to bed ____ am / pm

Fell Asleep ____ am / pm

Woke up ____ am / pm

Total Hours slept ______

# of Disruptions ______

Symptoms	Relief Attempts	Results Notes

Activity

- ☐ Walk - distance ______
- ☐ Physiotherapy
- ☐ Light Exercise
- ☐ Gym
- ☐ Housework
- ☐ ______
- ☐ ______

Medications taken

- ☐ Diabetes
- ☐ Blood Pressure
- ☐ Pain Management (Prescription)
- ☐ Pain (overcounter): ______
- ☐ Natural Therapies: ______
- ☐ Other: ______
- ☐ Other: ______

Medications

- ☐ No Change
- ☐ Dosage Changed
- ☐ from ______
- ☐ to ______
- ☐ Medication Changed
  - from ______
  - to ______

Daily Symptoms Tracker

Today,'s Dietary Intake

DAY

Drinks & Beverages

- ☐ Milk ☐ Juice ☐ Water
- ☐ Tea ☐ Coffee ☐ Soft / Energy Drink

Hydration

Breakfast

Blood Sugar: ____________
Blood Pressure: ____________
Temperature: ____________
Other: ____________

Lunch

Blood Sugar: ____________
Blood Pressure: ____________
Temperature: ____________
Other: ____________

Dinner

Blood Sugar: ____________
Blood Pressure: ____________
Temperature: ____________
Other: ____________

Snacks

Blood Sugar: ____________
Blood Pressure: ____________
Temperature: ____________
Other: ____________

- ☐ Fruit ☐ Vegetables ☐ Ginger Tea
- ☐ Grains & Cereals ☐ Fats

Weekly Summary

	Monday	Tuesday	Wednesday	Thursday	Friday	Saturday	Sunday
Pain							
Fatigue							
Weakness							
Stiffness							
Sleep (total Hours)							
# Disruptions							

Instructions:

Use the dots and dashes below to graph your ratings for the week - it helps to see things visually.

The bottom -- equals 0; the middle -- equals 5; and the top ◆ equals 10

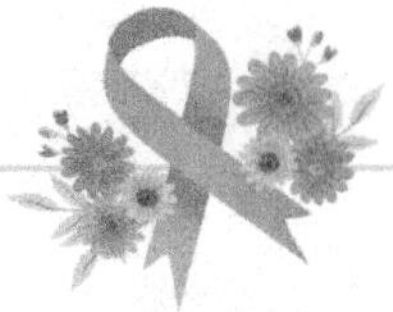

Weekly Summary

	Monday	Tuesday	Wednesday	Thursday	Friday	Saturday	Sunday
Anxiety							
Depression							
Stress							
Anger							
Brain Fog / Forgetfulness							

Daily Symptoms & Well-Being Tracker

DATE: ____ / ____ / ____

Today's Ratings

Pain ______ / 10
Fatigue ______ / 10
Weakness ______ / 10
Stiffness ______ / 10
General Mood ______

Anxiety ______ / 10
Depression ______ / 10
Stress ______ / 10
Anger ______ / 10

Sleep

Went to bed ____ am / pm
Fell Asleep ____ am / pm
Woke up ____ am / pm
Total Hours slept ______
# of Disruptions ______

Symptoms	Relief Attempts	Results Notes

Activity

- ☐ Walk - distance ______
- ☐ Physiotherapy
- ☐ Light Exercise
- ☐ Gym
- ☐ Housework
- ☐ ______
- ☐ ______

Medications taken

- ☐ Diabetes
- ☐ Blood Pressure
- ☐ Pain Management (Prescription)
- ☐ Pain (overcounter): ______
- ☐ Natural Therapies: ______
- ☐ Other: ______
- ☐ Other: ______

Medications

- ☐ No Change
- ☐ Dosage Changed
- ☐ from ______
- ☐ to ______
- ☐ Medication Changed

from ______
to ______

DAY

Today,'s Dietary Intake

Drinks & Beverages

- ☐ Milk
- ☐ Juice
- ☐ Water
- ☐ Tea
- ☐ Coffee
- ☐ Soft / Energy Drink

Hydration

Breakfast

____

____

____

Blood Sugar: ____________

Blood Pressure: ____________

Temperature: ____________

Other: ____________

Lunch

____

____

____

____

Blood Sugar: ____________

Blood Pressure: ____________

Temperature: ____________

Other: ____________

Dinner

____

____

____

____

____

Blood Sugar: ____________

Blood Pressure: ____________

Temperature: ____________

Other: ____________

Snacks

____

____

____

____

Blood Sugar: ____________

Blood Pressure: ____________

Temperature: ____________

Other: ____________

- ☐ Fruit
- ☐ Vegetables
- ☐ Ginger Tea
- ☐ Grains & Cereals
- ☐ Fats

Daily Symptoms & Well-Being Tracker

DATE: ____ / ____ / ____

Today's Ratings

Pain	______ / 10	Anxiety	______ / 10	Went to bed	____ am / pm
Fatigue	______ / 10	Depression	______ / 10	Fell Asleep	____ am / pm
Weakness	______ / 10	Stress	______ / 10	Woke up	____ am / pm
Stiffness	______ / 10	Anger	______ / 10	Total Hours slept	______
General Mood	______			# of Disruptions	______

Sleep

Symptoms	Relief Attempts	Results Notes

Activity

- ☐ Walk - distance ______
- ☐ Physiotherapy
- ☐ Light Exercise
- ☐ Gym
- ☐ Housework
- ☐ ______
- ☐ ______

Medications taken

- ☐ Diabetes
- ☐ Blood Pressure
- ☐ Pain Management (Prescription)
- ☐ Pain (overcounter): ______
- ☐ Natural Therapies: ______
- ☐ Other: ______
- ☐ Other: ______

Medications

- ☐ No Change
- ☐ Dosage Changed
- ☐ from ______
- ☐ to ______
- ☐ Medication Changed
- from ______
- to ______

DAY

Today,'s Dietary Intake

Drinks & Beverages

- ☐ Milk ☐ Juice ☐ Water
- ☐ Tea ☐ Coffee ☐ Soft / Energy Drink

Hydration

Breakfast

Blood Sugar: ______

Blood Pressure: ______

Temperature: ______

Other: ______

Lunch

Blood Sugar: ______

Blood Pressure: ______

Temperature: ______

Other: ______

Dinner

Blood Sugar: ______

Blood Pressure: ______

Temperature: ______

Other: ______

Snacks

Blood Sugar: ______

Blood Pressure: ______

Temperature: ______

Other: ______

- ☐ Fruit ☐ Vegetables ☐ Ginger Tea
- ☐ Grains & Cereals ☐ Fats

Daily Symptoms & Well-Being Tracker

DATE: ____ / ____ / ____

Today's Ratings

Pain	______ / 10	Anxiety	______ / 10	Went to bed	____ am / pm
Fatigue	______ / 10	Depression	______ / 10	Fell Asleep	____ am / pm
Weakness	______ / 10	Stress	______ / 10	Woke up	____ am / pm
Stiffness	______ / 10	Anger	______ / 10	Total Hours slept	______
General Mood	______			# of Disruptions	______

Sleep

Symptoms	Relief Attempts	Results Notes

Activity

- ☐ Walk - distance ______
- ☐ Physiotherapy
- ☐ Light Exercise
- ☐ Gym
- ☐ Housework
- ☐ ______
- ☐ ______

Medications taken

- ☐ Diabetes
- ☐ Blood Pressure
- ☐ Pain Management (Prescription)
- ☐ Pain (overcounter): ______
- ☐ Natural Therapies: ______
- ☐ Other: ______
- ☐ Other: ______

Medications

- ☐ No Change
- ☐ Dosage Changed
- ☐ from ______
- ☐ to ______
- ☐ Medication Changed
- from ______
- to ______

DAY

Today,'s Dietary Intake

Drinks & Beverages

- ☐ Milk
- ☐ Juice
- ☐ Water
- ☐ Tea
- ☐ Coffee
- ☐ Soft / Energy Drink

Hydration

☐ ☐ ☐ ☐ ☐ ☐ ☐

Breakfast

Blood Sugar: ______
Blood Pressure: ______
Temperature: ______
Other: ______

Lunch

Blood Sugar: ______
Blood Pressure: ______
Temperature: ______
Other: ______

Dinner

Blood Sugar: ______
Blood Pressure: ______
Temperature: ______
Other: ______

Snacks

Blood Sugar: ______
Blood Pressure: ______
Temperature: ______
Other: ______

- ☐ Fruit
- ☐ Vegetables
- ☐ Ginger Tea
- ☐ Grains & Cereals
- ☐ Fats

Daily Symptoms & Well-Being Tracker

DATE: ____ / ____ / ____

Today's Ratings

Pain	______ / 10	Anxiety	______ / 10	Went to bed	____ am / pm
Fatigue	______ / 10	Depression	______ / 10	Fell Asleep	____ am / pm
Weakness	______ / 10	Stress	______ / 10	Woke up	____ am / pm
Stiffness	______ / 10	Anger	______ / 10	Total Hours slept	______
General Mood	______			# of Disruptions	______

(The third column pair is headed **Sleep**.)

Symptoms	Relief Attempts	Results Notes

Activity

- ☐ Walk - distance ______
- ☐ Physiotherapy
- ☐ Light Exercise
- ☐ Gym
- ☐ Housework
- ☐ ______
- ☐ ______

Medications taken

- ☐ Diabetes
- ☐ Blood Pressure
- ☐ Pain Management (Prescription)
- ☐ Pain (overcounter): ______
- ☐ Natural Therapies: ______
- ☐ Other: ______
- ☐ Other: ______

Medications

- ☐ No Change
- ☐ Dosage Changed
- ☐ from ______
- ☐ to ______
- ☐ Medication Changed
- from ______
- to ______

DAY

Today,'s Dietary Intake

Drinks & Beverages

- ☐ Milk ☐ Juice ☐ Water
- ☐ Tea ☐ Coffee ☐ Soft / Energy Drink

Hydration

Breakfast

Blood Sugar: ______
Blood Pressure: ______
Temperature: ______
Other: ______

Lunch

Blood Sugar: ______
Blood Pressure: ______
Temperature: ______
Other: ______

Dinner

Blood Sugar: ______
Blood Pressure: ______
Temperature: ______
Other: ______

Snacks

Blood Sugar: ______
Blood Pressure: ______
Temperature: ______
Other: ______

- ☐ Fruit ☐ Vegetables ☐ Ginger Tea
- ☐ Grains & Cereals ☐ Fats

Daily Symptoms & Well-Being Tracker

DATE: ____ / ____ / ____

Today's Ratings

Pain	____ / 10	Anxiety	____ / 10
Fatigue	____ / 10	Depression	____ / 10
Weakness	____ / 10	Stress	____ / 10
Stiffness	____ / 10	Anger	____ / 10
General Mood	____		

Sleep

Went to bed	____ am / pm
Fell Asleep	____ am / pm
Woke up	____ am / pm
Total Hours slept	____
# of Disruptions	____

Symptoms	Relief Attempts	Results Notes

Activity

- ☐ Walk - distance ____
- ☐ Physiotherapy
- ☐ Light Exercise
- ☐ Gym
- ☐ Housework
- ☐ ____
- ☐ ____

Medications taken

- ☐ Diabetes
- ☐ Blood Pressure
- ☐ Pain Management (Prescription)
- ☐ Pain (overcounter): ____
- ☐ Natural Therapies: ____
- ☐ Other: ____
- ☐ Other: ____

Medications

- ☐ No Change
- ☐ Dosage Changed
- ☐ from ____
- ☐ to ____
- ☐ Medication Changed
  - from ____
  - to ____

DAY

Today,'s Dietary Intake

Drinks & Beverages

☐ Milk ☐ Juice ☐ Water

☐ Tea ☐ Coffee ☐ Soft / Energy Drink

Hydration

Breakfast

Blood Sugar: ______
Blood Pressure: ______
Temperature: ______
Other: ______

Lunch

Blood Sugar: ______
Blood Pressure: ______
Temperature: ______
Other: ______

Dinner

Blood Sugar: ______
Blood Pressure: ______
Temperature: ______
Other: ______

Snacks

Blood Sugar: ______
Blood Pressure: ______
Temperature: ______
Other: ______

☐ Fruit ☐ Vegetables ☐ Ginger Tea

☐ Grains & Cereals ☐ Fats

Daily Symptoms & Well-Being Tracker

DATE: ____ / ____ / ____

Today's Ratings

Pain	______ / 10	Anxiety	______ / 10	Went to bed	____ am / pm
Fatigue	______ / 10	Depression	______ / 10	Fell Asleep	____ am / pm
Weakness	______ / 10	Stress	______ / 10	Woke up	____ am / pm
Stiffness	______ / 10	Anger	______ / 10	Total Hours slept	______
General Mood	______			# of Disruptions	______

Sleep

Symptoms	Relief Attempts	Results Notes

Activity

- ☐ Walk - distance ______
- ☐ Physiotherapy
- ☐ Light Exercise
- ☐ Gym
- ☐ Housework
- ☐ ______
- ☐ ______

Medications taken

- ☐ Diabetes
- ☐ Blood Pressure
- ☐ Pain Management (Prescription)
- ☐ Pain (overcounter): ______
- ☐ Natural Therapies: ______
- ☐ Other: ______
- ☐ Other: ______

Medications

- ☐ No Change
- ☐ Dosage Changed
- ☐ from ______
- ☐ to ______
- ☐ Medication Changed
  - from ______
  - to ______

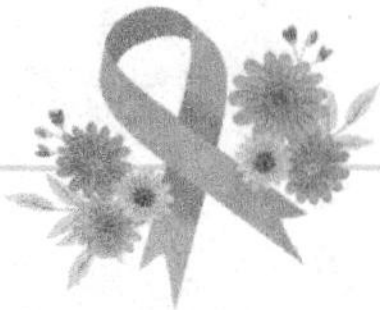

DAY

Today,'s Dietary Intake

Drinks & Beverages

- ☐ Milk
- ☐ Juice
- ☐ Water
- ☐ Tea
- ☐ Coffee
- ☐ Soft / Energy Drink

Hydration

Breakfast

Blood Sugar: ______
Blood Pressure: ______
Temperature: ______
Other: ______

Lunch

Blood Sugar: ______
Blood Pressure: ______
Temperature: ______
Other: ______

Dinner

Blood Sugar: ______
Blood Pressure: ______
Temperature: ______
Other: ______

Snacks

Blood Sugar: ______
Blood Pressure: ______
Temperature: ______
Other: ______

- ☐ Fruit
- ☐ Vegetables
- ☐ Ginger Tea
- ☐ Grains & Cereals
- ☐ Fats

Daily Symptoms & Well-Being Tracker

DATE: ____ / ____ / ____

Today's Ratings

Pain	____ / 10	Anxiety	____ / 10
Fatigue	____ / 10	Depression	____ / 10
Weakness	____ / 10	Stress	____ / 10
Stiffness	____ / 10	Anger	____ / 10
General Mood	____		

Sleep

Went to bed	____ am / pm
Fell Asleep	____ am / pm
Woke up	____ am / pm
Total Hours slept	____
# of Disruptions	____

Symptoms	Relief Attempts	Results Notes

Activity

- ☐ Walk - distance ____
- ☐ Physiotherapy
- ☐ Light Exercise
- ☐ Gym
- ☐ Housework
- ☐ ____
- ☐ ____

Medications taken

- ☐ Diabetes
- ☐ Blood Pressure
- ☐ Pain Management (Prescription)
- ☐ Pain (overcounter): ____
- ☐ Natural Therapies: ____
- ☐ Other: ____
- ☐ Other: ____

Medications

- ☐ No Change
- ☐ Dosage Changed
- ☐ from ____
- ☐ to ____
- ☐ Medication Changed
  - from ____
  - to ____

Today,'s Dietary Intake

DAY

Drinks & Beverages

- ☐ Milk ☐ Juice ☐ Water
- ☐ Tea ☐ Coffee ☐ Soft / Energy Drink

Hydration

Meal	Readings
Breakfast	Blood Sugar: ____ Blood Pressure: ____ Temperature: ____ Other: ____
Lunch	Blood Sugar: ____ Blood Pressure: ____ Temperature: ____ Other: ____
Dinner	Blood Sugar: ____ Blood Pressure: ____ Temperature: ____ Other: ____
Snacks	Blood Sugar: ____ Blood Pressure: ____ Temperature: ____ Other: ____

- ☐ Fruit ☐ Vegetables ☐ Ginger Tea
- ☐ Grains & Cereals ☐ Fats

Weekly Summary

	Monday	Tuesday	Wednesday	Thursday	Friday	Saturday	Sunday
Pain							
Fatigue							
Weakness							
Stiffness							
Sleep (total Hours)							
# Disruptions							

Instructions:

Use the dots and dashes below to graph your ratings for the week - it helps to see things visually.

The bottom -- equals 0; the middle -- equals 5; and the top ◆ equals 10

Weekly Summary

	Monday	Tuesday	Wednesday	Thursday	Friday	Saturday	Sunday
Anxiety							
Depression							
Stress							
Anger							
Brain Fog / Forgetfulness							

Daily Symptoms & Well-Being Tracker

DATE: ____ / ____ / ____

Today's Ratings

Pain	____ / 10	Anxiety	____ / 10	Went to bed	____ am / pm
Fatigue	____ / 10	Depression	____ / 10	Fell Asleep	____ am / pm
Weakness	____ / 10	Stress	____ / 10	Woke up	____ am / pm
Stiffness	____ / 10	Anger	____ / 10	Total Hours slept	____
General Mood	____			# of Disruptions	____

Sleep

Symptoms	Relief Attempts	Results Notes

Activity

- ☐ Walk - distance ____
- ☐ Physiotherapy
- ☐ Light Exercise
- ☐ Gym
- ☐ Housework
- ☐ ____
- ☐ ____

Medications taken

- ☐ Diabetes
- ☐ Blood Pressure
- ☐ Pain Management (Prescription)
- ☐ Pain (overcounter): ____
- ☐ Natural Therapies: ____
- ☐ Other: ____
- ☐ Other: ____

Medications

- ☐ No Change
- ☐ Dosage Changed
- ☐ from ____
- ☐ to ____
- ☐ Medication Changed
  - from ____
  - to ____

Today,'s Dietary Intake

DAY

Drinks & Beverages

- ☐ Milk ☐ Juice ☐ Water
- ☐ Tea ☐ Coffee ☐ Soft / Energy Drink

Hydration

☐ ☐ ☐ ☐ ☐ ☐ ☐

Breakfast	Blood Sugar: ______
______	Blood Pressure: ______
______	Temperature: ______
______	Other: ______
Lunch	
______	Blood Sugar: ______
______	Blood Pressure: ______
______	Temperature: ______
______	Other: ______
Dinner	
______	Blood Sugar: ______
______	Blood Pressure: ______
______	Temperature: ______
______	Other: ______
______	
Snacks	
______	Blood Sugar: ______
______	Blood Pressure: ______
______	Temperature: ______
______	Other: ______

- ☐ Fruit ☐ Vegetables ☐ Ginger Tea
- ☐ Grains & Cereals ☐ Fats

Daily Symptoms & Well-Being Tracker

DATE: ____ / ____ / ____

Today's Ratings

Pain	____ / 10	Anxiety	____ / 10
Fatigue	____ / 10	Depression	____ / 10
Weakness	____ / 10	Stress	____ / 10
Stiffness	____ / 10	Anger	____ / 10
General Mood	____		

Sleep

Went to bed	____ am / pm
Fell Asleep	____ am / pm
Woke up	____ am / pm
Total Hours slept	____
# of Disruptions	____

Symptoms	Relief Attempts	Results Notes

Activity

- ☐ Walk - distance ____
- ☐ Physiotherapy
- ☐ Light Exercise
- ☐ Gym
- ☐ Housework
- ☐ ____
- ☐ ____

Medications taken

- ☐ Diabetes
- ☐ Blood Pressure
- ☐ Pain Management (Prescription)
- ☐ Pain (overcounter): ____
- ☐ Natural Therapies: ____
- ☐ Other: ____
- ☐ Other: ____

Medications

- ☐ No Change
- ☐ Dosage Changed
- ☐ from ____
- ☐ to ____
- ☐ Medication Changed
- from ____
- to ____

DAY

Today,'s Dietary Intake

Drinks & Beverages

- ☐ Milk
- ☐ Juice
- ☐ Water
- ☐ Tea
- ☐ Coffee
- ☐ Soft / Energy Drink

Hydration

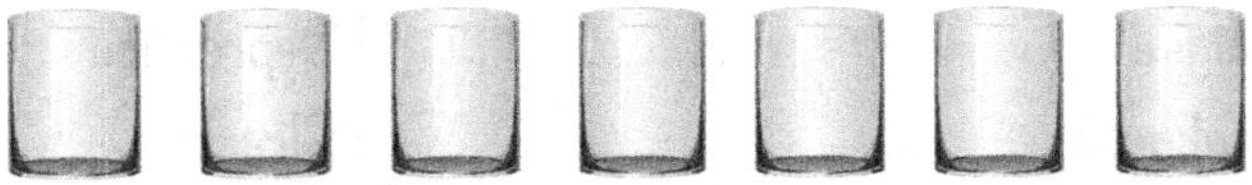

Breakfast	
	Blood Sugar:
	Blood Pressure:
	Temperature:
	Other:

Lunch	
	Blood Sugar:
	Blood Pressure:
	Temperature:
	Other:

Dinner	
	Blood Sugar:
	Blood Pressure:
	Temperature:
	Other:

Snacks	
	Blood Sugar:
	Blood Pressure:
	Temperature:
	Other:

- ☐ Fruit
- ☐ Vegetables
- ☐ Ginger Tea
- ☐ Grains & Cereals
- ☐ Fats

Daily Symptoms & Well-Being Tracker

DATE: ____ / ____ / ____

Today's Ratings

Pain ________ / 10
Fatigue ________ / 10
Weakness ________ / 10
Stiffness ________ / 10
General Mood ________

Anxiety ________ / 10
Depression ________ / 10
Stress ________ / 10
Anger ________ / 10

Sleep

Went to bed ____ am / pm
Fell Asleep ____ am / pm
Woke up ____ am / pm
Total Hours slept ________
# of Disruptions ________

Symptoms	Relief Attempts	Results Notes

Activity

- ☐ Walk - distance ________
- ☐ Physiotherapy
- ☐ Light Exercise
- ☐ Gym
- ☐ Housework
- ☐ ________
- ☐ ________

Medications taken

- ☐ Diabetes
- ☐ Blood Pressure
- ☐ Pain Management (Prescription)
- ☐ Pain (overcounter): ________
- ☐ Natural Therapies: ________
- ☐ Other: ________
- ☐ Other: ________

Medications

- ☐ No Change
- ☐ Dosage Changed
- ☐ from ________
- ☐ to ________
- ☐ Medication Changed

from ________

to ________

DAY

Today,'s Dietary Intake

Drinks & Beverages

- ☐ Milk
- ☐ Juice
- ☐ Water
- ☐ Tea
- ☐ Coffee
- ☐ Soft / Energy Drink

Hydration

Breakfast	Blood Sugar: ____ Blood Pressure: ____ Temperature: ____ Other: ____
Lunch	Blood Sugar: ____ Blood Pressure: ____ Temperature: ____ Other: ____
Dinner	Blood Sugar: ____ Blood Pressure: ____ Temperature: ____ Other: ____
Snacks	Blood Sugar: ____ Blood Pressure: ____ Temperature: ____ Other: ____

- ☐ Fruit
- ☐ Vegetables
- ☐ Ginger Tea
- ☐ Grains & Cereals
- ☐ Fats

Daily Symptoms & Well-Being Tracker

DATE: ____ / ____ / ____

Today's Ratings

Pain	______ / 10	Anxiety	______ / 10	Went to bed	____ am / pm
Fatigue	______ / 10	Depression	______ / 10	Fell Asleep	____ am / pm
Weakness	______ / 10	Stress	______ / 10	Woke up	____ am / pm
Stiffness	______ / 10	Anger	______ / 10	Total Hours slept	______
General Mood	______			# of Disruptions	______

Sleep

Symptoms	Relief Attempts	Results Notes

Activity

- ☐ Walk - distance ______
- ☐ Physiotherapy
- ☐ Light Exercise
- ☐ Gym
- ☐ Housework
- ☐ ______
- ☐ ______

Medications taken

- ☐ Diabetes
- ☐ Blood Pressure
- ☐ Pain Management (Prescription)
- ☐ Pain (overcounter): ______
- ☐ Natural Therapies: ______
- ☐ Other: ______
- ☐ Other: ______

Medications

- ☐ No Change
- ☐ Dosage Changed
- ☐ from ______
- ☐ to ______
- ☐ Medication Changed
- from ______
- to ______

Today,'s Dietary Intake

DAY

Drinks & Beverages

- ☐ Milk ☐ Juice ☐ Water
- ☐ Tea ☐ Coffee ☐ Soft / Energy Drink

Hydration

Breakfast

Blood Sugar: ____
Blood Pressure: ____
Temperature: ____
Other: ____

Lunch

Blood Sugar: ____
Blood Pressure: ____
Temperature: ____
Other: ____

Dinner

Blood Sugar: ____
Blood Pressure: ____
Temperature: ____
Other: ____

Snacks

Blood Sugar: ____
Blood Pressure: ____
Temperature: ____
Other: ____

- ☐ Fruit ☐ Vegetables ☐ Ginger Tea
- ☐ Grains & Cereals ☐ Fats

Daily Symptoms & Well-Being Tracker

DATE: ____ / ____ / ____

Today's Ratings

Pain	______ / 10	Anxiety	______ / 10		
Fatigue	______ / 10	Depression	______ / 10		
Weakness	______ / 10	Stress	______ / 10		
Stiffness	______ / 10	Anger	______ / 10		
General Mood	______				

Sleep

Went to bed	____ am / pm
Fell Asleep	____ am / pm
Woke up	____ am / pm
Total Hours slept	______
# of Disruptions	______

Symptoms	Relief Attempts	Results Notes

Activity

- ☐ Walk - distance ______
- ☐ Physiotherapy
- ☐ Light Exercise
- ☐ Gym
- ☐ Housework
- ☐ ______
- ☐ ______

Medications taken

- ☐ Diabetes
- ☐ Blood Pressure
- ☐ Pain Management (Prescription)
- ☐ Pain (overcounter): ______
- ☐ Natural Therapies: ______
- ☐ Other: ______
- ☐ Other: ______

Medications

- ☐ No Change
- ☐ Dosage Changed
- ☐ from ______
- ☐ to ______
- ☐ Medication Changed
- from ______
- to ______

Daily Symptoms Tracker

Today,'s Dietary Intake

DAY

Drinks & Beverages

- ☐ Milk
- ☐ Juice
- ☐ Water
- ☐ Tea
- ☐ Coffee
- ☐ Soft / Energy Drink

Hydration

Breakfast

Blood Sugar: ____________
Blood Pressure: ____________
Temperature: ____________
Other: ____________

Lunch

Blood Sugar: ____________
Blood Pressure: ____________
Temperature: ____________
Other: ____________

Dinner

Blood Sugar: ____________
Blood Pressure: ____________
Temperature: ____________
Other: ____________

Snacks

Blood Sugar: ____________
Blood Pressure: ____________
Temperature: ____________
Other: ____________

- ☐ Fruit
- ☐ Vegetables
- ☐ Ginger Tea
- ☐ Grains & Cereals
- ☐ Fats

Daily Symptoms & Well-Being Tracker

DATE: ____ / ____ / ____

Today's Ratings

Pain	______ / 10	Anxiety	______ / 10	Went to bed	____ am / pm
Fatigue	______ / 10	Depression	______ / 10	Fell Asleep	____ am / pm
Weakness	______ / 10	Stress	______ / 10	Woke up	____ am / pm
Stiffness	______ / 10	Anger	______ / 10	Total Hours slept	______
General Mood	______			# of Disruptions	______

(Sleep)

Symptoms	Relief Attempts	Results Notes

Activity

- ☐ Walk - distance ______
- ☐ Physiotherapy
- ☐ Light Exercise
- ☐ Gym
- ☐ Housework
- ☐ ______
- ☐ ______

Medications taken

- ☐ Diabetes
- ☐ Blood Pressure
- ☐ Pain Management (Prescription)
- ☐ Pain (overcounter): ______
- ☐ Natural Therapies: ______
- ☐ Other: ______
- ☐ Other: ______

Medications

- ☐ No Change
- ☐ Dosage Changed
- ☐ from ______
- ☐ to ______
- ☐ Medication Changed
  - from ______
  - to ______

Today,'s Dietary Intake

DAY

Drinks & Beverages

- ☐ Milk ☐ Juice ☐ Water
- ☐ Tea ☐ Coffee ☐ Soft / Energy Drink

Hydration

☐ ☐ ☐ ☐ ☐ ☐ ☐

Meal	Readings
Breakfast ______ ______ ______	Blood Sugar: ______ Blood Pressure: ______ Temperature: ______ Other: ______
Lunch ______ ______ ______ ______	Blood Sugar: ______ Blood Pressure: ______ Temperature: ______ Other: ______
Dinner ______ ______ ______ ______ ______	Blood Sugar: ______ Blood Pressure: ______ Temperature: ______ Other: ______
Snacks ______ ______ ______ ______	Blood Sugar: ______ Blood Pressure: ______ Temperature: ______ Other: ______

- ☐ Fruit ☐ Vegetables ☐ Ginger Tea
- ☐ Grains & Cereals ☐ Fats

Daily Symptoms & Well-Being Tracker

DATE: ____ / ____ / ____

Today's Ratings

Pain	______ / 10	Anxiety	______ / 10
Fatigue	______ / 10	Depression	______ / 10
Weakness	______ / 10	Stress	______ / 10
Stiffness	______ / 10	Anger	______ / 10
General Mood	______		

Sleep

Went to bed	____ am / pm
Fell Asleep	____ am / pm
Woke up	____ am / pm
Total Hours slept	______
# of Disruptions	______

Symptoms	Relief Attempts	Results Notes

Activity

- ☐ Walk - distance ______
- ☐ Physiotherapy
- ☐ Light Exercise
- ☐ Gym
- ☐ Housework
- ☐ ______
- ☐ ______

Medications taken

- ☐ Diabetes
- ☐ Blood Pressure
- ☐ Pain Management (Prescription)
- ☐ Pain (overcounter): ______
- ☐ Natural Therapies: ______
- ☐ Other: ______
- ☐ Other: ______

Medications

- ☐ No Change
- ☐ Dosage Changed
- ☐ from ______
- ☐ to ______
- ☐ Medication Changed
  - from ______
  - to ______

Today,'s Dietary Intake

DAY

Drinks & Beverages

- ☐ Milk
- ☐ Juice
- ☐ Water
- ☐ Tea
- ☐ Coffee
- ☐ Soft / Energy Drink

Hydration

Breakfast

Blood Sugar: ______
Blood Pressure: ______
Temperature: ______
Other: ______

Lunch

Blood Sugar: ______
Blood Pressure: ______
Temperature: ______
Other: ______

Dinner

Blood Sugar: ______
Blood Pressure: ______
Temperature: ______
Other: ______

Snacks

Blood Sugar: ______
Blood Pressure: ______
Temperature: ______
Other: ______

- ☐ Fruit
- ☐ Vegetables
- ☐ Ginger Tea
- ☐ Grains & Cereals
- ☐ Fats

Weekly Summary

	Monday	Tuesday	Wednesday	Thursday	Friday	Saturday	Sunday
Pain							
Fatigue							
Weakness							
Stiffness							
Sleep (total Hours)							
# Disruptions							

Instructions:

Use the dots and dashes below to graph your ratings for the week – it helps to see things visually.

The bottom -- equals 0; the middle -- equals 5; and the top ◆ equals 10

Weekly Summary

	Monday	Tuesday	Wednesday	Thursday	Friday	Saturday	Sunday
Anxiety							
Depression							
Stress							
Anger							
Brain Fog / Forgetfulness							

Daily Symptoms & Well-Being Tracker

DATE: ____ / ____ / ____

Today's Ratings

Pain ________ / 10
Fatigue ________ / 10
Weakness ________ / 10
Stiffness ________ / 10
General Mood ____________

Anxiety ________ / 10
Depression ________ / 10
Stress ________ / 10
Anger ________ / 10

Sleep

Went to bed _____ am / pm
Fell Asleep _____ am / pm
Woke up _____ am / pm
Total Hours slept ____________
# of Disruptions ____________

Symptoms	Relief Attempts	Results Notes

Activity

- ☐ Walk - distance ________
- ☐ Physiotherapy
- ☐ Light Exercise
- ☐ Gym
- ☐ Housework
- ☐ ____________
- ☐ ____________

Medications taken

- ☐ Diabetes
- ☐ Blood Pressure
- ☐ Pain Management (Prescription)
- ☐ Pain (overcounter): ____________
- ☐ Natural Therapies: ____________
- ☐ Other: ____________
- ☐ Other: ____________

Medications

- ☐ No Change
- ☐ Dosage Changed
- ☐ from ____________
- ☐ to ____________
- ☐ Medication Changed
  from ____________
  to ____________

Daily Symptoms Tracker

Today.'s Dietary Intake

DAY

Drinks & Beverages

- ☐ Milk
- ☐ Juice
- ☐ Water
- ☐ Tea
- ☐ Coffee
- ☐ Soft / Energy Drink

Hydration

Breakfast

Blood Sugar: ______

Blood Pressure: ______

Temperature: ______

Other: ______

Lunch

Blood Sugar: ______

Blood Pressure: ______

Temperature: ______

Other: ______

Dinner

Blood Sugar: ______

Blood Pressure: ______

Temperature: ______

Other: ______

Snacks

Blood Sugar: ______

Blood Pressure: ______

Temperature: ______

Other: ______

- ☐ Fruit
- ☐ Vegetables
- ☐ Ginger Tea
- ☐ Grains & Cereals
- ☐ Fats

Daily Symptoms & Well-Being Tracker

DATE: ____ / ____ / ____

Today's Ratings

Pain	______ / 10	Anxiety	______ / 10	Went to bed	____ am / pm
Fatigue	______ / 10	Depression	______ / 10	Fell Asleep	____ am / pm
Weakness	______ / 10	Stress	______ / 10	Woke up	____ am / pm
Stiffness	______ / 10	Anger	______ / 10	Total Hours slept	______
General Mood	______			# of Disruptions	______

Symptoms	Relief Attempts	Results Notes

Activity

- ☐ Walk - distance ______
- ☐ Physiotherapy
- ☐ Light Exercise
- ☐ Gym
- ☐ Housework
- ☐ ______
- ☐ ______

Medications taken

- ☐ Diabetes
- ☐ Blood Pressure
- ☐ Pain Management (Prescription)
- ☐ Pain (overcounter): ______
- ☐ Natural Therapies: ______
- ☐ Other: ______
- ☐ Other: ______

Medications

- ☐ No Change
- ☐ Dosage Changed
- ☐ from ______
- ☐ to ______
- ☐ Medication Changed
  - from ______
  - to ______

DAY

Today,'s Dietary Intake

Drinks & Beverages

- ☐ Milk ☐ Juice ☐ Water
- ☐ Tea ☐ Coffee ☐ Soft / Energy Drink

Hydration

Breakfast

Blood Sugar: ________
Blood Pressure: ________
Temperature: ________
Other: ________

Lunch

Blood Sugar: ________
Blood Pressure: ________
Temperature: ________
Other: ________

Dinner

Blood Sugar: ________
Blood Pressure: ________
Temperature: ________
Other: ________

Snacks

Blood Sugar: ________
Blood Pressure: ________
Temperature: ________
Other: ________

- ☐ Fruit ☐ Vegetables ☐ Ginger Tea
- ☐ Grains & Cereals ☐ Fats

Daily Symptoms & Well-Being Tracker

DATE: ____ / ____ / ____

Today's Ratings

Pain	______ / 10	Anxiety	______ / 10	Went to bed	____ am / pm
Fatigue	______ / 10	Depression	______ / 10	Fell Asleep	____ am / pm
Weakness	______ / 10	Stress	______ / 10	Woke up	____ am / pm
Stiffness	______ / 10	Anger	______ / 10	Total Hours slept	______
General Mood	______			# of Disruptions	______

Symptoms	Relief Attempts	Results Notes

Activity

- ☐ Walk - distance ______
- ☐ Physiotherapy
- ☐ Light Exercise
- ☐ Gym
- ☐ Housework
- ☐ ______
- ☐ ______

Medications taken

- ☐ Diabetes
- ☐ Blood Pressure
- ☐ Pain Management (Prescription)
- ☐ Pain (overcounter): ______
- ☐ Natural Therapies: ______
- ☐ Other: ______
- ☐ Other: ______

Medications

- ☐ No Change
- ☐ Dosage Changed
- ☐ from ______
- ☐ to ______
- ☐ Medication Changed
  - from ______
  - to ______

DAY

Today,'s Dietary Intake

Drinks & Beverages

- ☐ Milk ☐ Juice ☐ Water
- ☐ Tea ☐ Coffee ☐ Soft / Energy Drink

Hydration

Breakfast

Blood Sugar:
Blood Pressure:
Temperature:
Other:

Lunch

Blood Sugar:
Blood Pressure:
Temperature:
Other:

Dinner

Blood Sugar:
Blood Pressure:
Temperature:
Other:

Snacks

Blood Sugar:
Blood Pressure:
Temperature:
Other:

- ☐ Fruit ☐ Vegetables ☐ Ginger Tea
- ☐ Grains & Cereals ☐ Fats

Daily Symptoms & Well-Being Tracker

DATE: ____ / ____ / ____

Today's Ratings

Pain	______ / 10	Anxiety	______ / 10	Went to bed	____ am / pm
Fatigue	______ / 10	Depression	______ / 10	Fell Asleep	____ am / pm
Weakness	______ / 10	Stress	______ / 10	Woke up	____ am / pm
Stiffness	______ / 10	Anger	______ / 10	Total Hours slept	______
General Mood	______			# of Disruptions	______

Sleep

Symptoms	Relief Attempts	Results Notes

Activity

- ☐ Walk - distance ______
- ☐ Physiotherapy
- ☐ Light Exercise
- ☐ Gym
- ☐ Housework
- ☐ ______
- ☐ ______

Medications taken

- ☐ Diabetes
- ☐ Blood Pressure
- ☐ Pain Management (Prescription)
- ☐ Pain (overcounter): ______
- ☐ Natural Therapies: ______
- ☐ Other: ______
- ☐ Other: ______

Medications

- ☐ No Change
- ☐ Dosage Changed
- ☐ from ______
- ☐ to ______
- ☐ Medication Changed
- from ______
- to ______

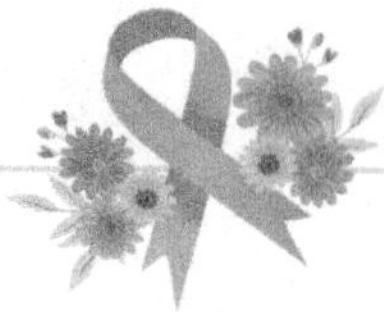

DAY

Today,'s Dietary Intake

Drinks & Beverages

- ☐ Milk ☐ Juice ☐ Water
- ☐ Tea ☐ Coffee ☐ Soft / Energy Drink

Hydration

Breakfast __________ __________ __________	Blood Sugar: ______ Blood Pressure: ______ Temperature: ______ Other: ______
Lunch __________ __________ __________ __________	Blood Sugar: ______ Blood Pressure: ______ Temperature: ______ Other: ______
Dinner __________ __________ __________ __________ __________	Blood Sugar: ______ Blood Pressure: ______ Temperature: ______ Other: ______
Snacks __________ __________ __________ __________	Blood Sugar: ______ Blood Pressure: ______ Temperature: ______ Other: ______

- ☐ Fruit ☐ Vegetables ☐ Ginger Tea
- ☐ Grains & Cereals ☐ Fats

Daily Symptoms & Well-Being Tracker

DATE: ____ / ____ / ____

Today's Ratings

Pain ________ / 10
Fatigue ________ / 10
Weakness ________ / 10
Stiffness ________ / 10
General Mood ________

Anxiety ________ / 10
Depression ________ / 10
Stress ________ / 10
Anger ________ / 10

Sleep

Went to bed ____ am / pm
Fell Asleep ____ am / pm
Woke up ____ am / pm
Total Hours slept ________
# of Disruptions ________

Symptoms	Relief Attempts	Results Notes

Activity

- ☐ Walk - distance ________
- ☐ Physiotherapy
- ☐ Light Exercise
- ☐ Gym
- ☐ Housework
- ☐ ________
- ☐ ________

Medications taken

- ☐ Diabetes
- ☐ Blood Pressure
- ☐ Pain Management (Prescription)
- ☐ Pain (overcounter): ________
- ☐ Natural Therapies: ________
- ☐ Other: ________
- ☐ Other: ________

Medications

- ☐ No Change
- ☐ Dosage Changed
- ☐ from ________
- ☐ to ________
- ☐ Medication Changed
  from ________
  to ________

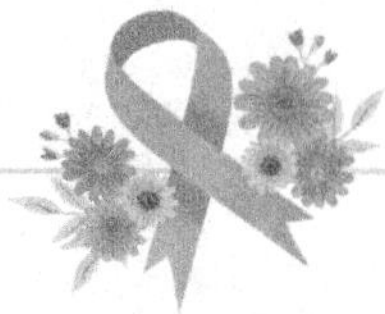

DAY

Today,'s Dietary Intake

Drinks & Beverages

- ☐ Milk ☐ Juice ☐ Water
- ☐ Tea ☐ Coffee ☐ Soft / Energy Drink

Hydration

Breakfast

Blood Sugar: ____________
Blood Pressure: ____________
Temperature: ____________
Other: ____________

Lunch

Blood Sugar: ____________
Blood Pressure: ____________
Temperature: ____________
Other: ____________

Dinner

Blood Sugar: ____________
Blood Pressure: ____________
Temperature: ____________
Other: ____________

Snacks

Blood Sugar: ____________
Blood Pressure: ____________
Temperature: ____________
Other: ____________

- ☐ Fruit ☐ Vegetables ☐ Ginger Tea
- ☐ Grains & Cereals ☐ Fats

Daily Symptoms & Well-Being Tracker

DATE: ____ / ____ / ____

Today's Ratings

Pain	______ / 10	Anxiety	______ / 10	Went to bed	____ am / pm
Fatigue	______ / 10	Depression	______ / 10	Fell Asleep	____ am / pm
Weakness	______ / 10	Stress	______ / 10	Woke up	____ am / pm
Stiffness	______ / 10	Anger	______ / 10	Total Hours slept	______
General Mood	______			# of Disruptions	______

Symptoms	Relief Attempts	Results Notes

Activity

- ☐ Walk - distance ______
- ☐ Physiotherapy
- ☐ Light Exercise
- ☐ Gym
- ☐ Housework
- ☐ ______
- ☐ ______

Medications taken

- ☐ Diabetes
- ☐ Blood Pressure
- ☐ Pain Management (Prescription)
- ☐ Pain (overcounter): ______
- ☐ Natural Therapies: ______
- ☐ Other: ______
- ☐ Other: ______

Medications

- ☐ No Change
- ☐ Dosage Changed
- ☐ from ______
- ☐ to ______
- ☐ Medication Changed
  - from ______
  - to ______

DAY

Today.'s Dietary Intake

Drinks & Beverages

- ☐ Milk ☐ Juice ☐ Water
- ☐ Tea ☐ Coffee ☐ Soft / Energy Drink

Hydration

Breakfast

Blood Sugar:
Blood Pressure:
Temperature:
Other:

Lunch

Blood Sugar:
Blood Pressure:
Temperature:
Other:

Dinner

Blood Sugar:
Blood Pressure:
Temperature:
Other:

Snacks

Blood Sugar:
Blood Pressure:
Temperature:
Other:

- ☐ Fruit ☐ Vegetables ☐ Ginger Tea
- ☐ Grains & Cereals ☐ Fats

Daily Symptoms & Well-Being Tracker

DATE: ____ / ____ / ____

Today's Ratings

Pain	______ / 10	Anxiety	______ / 10
Fatigue	______ / 10	Depression	______ / 10
Weakness	______ / 10	Stress	______ / 10
Stiffness	______ / 10	Anger	______ / 10
General Mood	______		

Sleep

Went to bed	____ am / pm
Fell Asleep	____ am / pm
Woke up	____ am / pm
Total Hours slept	______
# of Disruptions	______

Symptoms	Relief Attempts	Results Notes

Activity

- ☐ Walk - distance ______
- ☐ Physiotherapy
- ☐ Light Exercise
- ☐ Gym
- ☐ Housework
- ☐ ______
- ☐ ______

Medications taken

- ☐ Diabetes
- ☐ Blood Pressure
- ☐ Pain Management (Prescription)
- ☐ Pain (overcounter): ______
- ☐ Natural Therapies: ______
- ☐ Other: ______
- ☐ Other: ______

Medications

- ☐ No Change
- ☐ Dosage Changed
- ☐ from ______
- ☐ to ______
- ☐ Medication Changed
  - from ______
  - to ______

DAY

Today,'s Dietary Intake

Drinks & Beverages

- ☐ Milk ☐ Juice ☐ Water
- ☐ Tea ☐ Coffee ☐ Soft / Energy Drink

Hydration

Breakfast

Blood Sugar: ______
Blood Pressure: ______
Temperature: ______
Other: ______

Lunch

Blood Sugar: ______
Blood Pressure: ______
Temperature: ______
Other: ______

Dinner

Blood Sugar: ______
Blood Pressure: ______
Temperature: ______
Other: ______

Snacks

Blood Sugar: ______
Blood Pressure: ______
Temperature: ______
Other: ______

- ☐ Fruit ☐ Vegetables ☐ Ginger Tea
- ☐ Grains & Cereals ☐ Fats

Weekly Summary

	Monday	Tuesday	Wednesday	Thursday	Friday	Saturday	Sunday
Pain							
Fatigue							
Weakness							
Stiffness							
Sleep (total Hours)							
# Disruptions							

Instructions:

Use the dots and dashes below to graph your ratings for the week – it helps to see things visually.

The bottom -- equals 0; the middle -- equals 5; and the top ◆ equals 10

Weekly Summary

	Monday	Tuesday	Wednesday	Thursday	Friday	Saturday	Sunday
Anxiety							
Depression							
Stress							
Anger							
Brain Fog / Forgetfulness							

Daily Symptoms & Well-Being Tracker

DATE: ____ / ____ / ____

Today's Ratings

Pain	______ / 10	Anxiety	______ / 10	Went to bed	____ am / pm
Fatigue	______ / 10	Depression	______ / 10	Fell Asleep	____ am / pm
Weakness	______ / 10	Stress	______ / 10	Woke up	____ am / pm
Stiffness	______ / 10	Anger	______ / 10	Total Hours slept	______
General Mood	______			# of Disruptions	______

(Sleep)

Symptoms	Relief Attempts	Results Notes

Activity

- ☐ Walk - distance ______
- ☐ Physiotherapy
- ☐ Light Exercise
- ☐ Gym
- ☐ Housework
- ☐ ______
- ☐ ______

Medications taken

- ☐ Diabetes
- ☐ Blood Pressure
- ☐ Pain Management (Prescription)
- ☐ Pain (overcounter): ______
- ☐ Natural Therapies: ______
- ☐ Other: ______
- ☐ Other: ______

Medications

- ☐ No Change
- ☐ Dosage Changed
- ☐ from ______
- ☐ to ______
- ☐ Medication Changed
  - from ______
  - to ______

DAY

Today,'s Dietary Intake

Drinks & Beverages

- ☐ Milk
- ☐ Juice
- ☐ Water
- ☐ Tea
- ☐ Coffee
- ☐ Soft / Energy Drink

Hydration

Breakfast

Blood Sugar: ______
Blood Pressure: ______
Temperature: ______
Other: ______

Lunch

Blood Sugar: ______
Blood Pressure: ______
Temperature: ______
Other: ______

Dinner

Blood Sugar: ______
Blood Pressure: ______
Temperature: ______
Other: ______

Snacks

Blood Sugar: ______
Blood Pressure: ______
Temperature: ______
Other: ______

- ☐ Fruit
- ☐ Vegetables
- ☐ Ginger Tea
- ☐ Grains & Cereals
- ☐ Fats

Daily Symptoms & Well-Being Tracker

DATE: ____ / ____ / ____

Today's Ratings

Pain	______ / 10	Anxiety	______ / 10	Went to bed	____ am / pm
Fatigue	______ / 10	Depression	______ / 10	Fell Asleep	____ am / pm
Weakness	______ / 10	Stress	______ / 10	Woke up	____ am / pm
Stiffness	______ / 10	Anger	______ / 10	Total Hours slept	______
General Mood	______			# of Disruptions	______

Sleep

Symptoms	Relief Attempts	Results Notes

Activity

- ☐ Walk - distance ______
- ☐ Physiotherapy
- ☐ Light Exercise
- ☐ Gym
- ☐ Housework
- ☐ ______
- ☐ ______

Medications taken

- ☐ Diabetes
- ☐ Blood Pressure
- ☐ Pain Management (Prescription)
- ☐ Pain (overcounter): ______
- ☐ Natural Therapies: ______
- ☐ Other: ______
- ☐ Other: ______

Medications

- ☐ No Change
- ☐ Dosage Changed
- ☐ from ______
- ☐ to ______
- ☐ Medication Changed
  - from ______
  - to ______

DAY

Today,'s Dietary Intake

Drinks & Beverages

☐ Milk ☐ Juice ☐ Water

☐ Tea ☐ Coffee ☐ Soft / Energy Drink

Hydration

Breakfast

Blood Sugar: ________

Blood Pressure: ________

Temperature: ________

Other: ________

Lunch

Blood Sugar: ________

Blood Pressure: ________

Temperature: ________

Other: ________

Dinner

Blood Sugar: ________

Blood Pressure: ________

Temperature: ________

Other: ________

Snacks

Blood Sugar: ________

Blood Pressure: ________

Temperature: ________

Other: ________

☐ Fruit ☐ Vegetables ☐ Ginger Tea

☐ Grains & Cereals ☐ Fats

Daily Symptoms & Well-Being Tracker

DATE: ____ / ____ / ____

Today's Ratings

Pain	______ / 10
Fatigue	______ / 10
Weakness	______ / 10
Stiffness	______ / 10
General Mood	______

Anxiety	______ / 10
Depression	______ / 10
Stress	______ / 10
Anger	______ / 10

Sleep

Went to bed	____ am / pm
Fell Asleep	____ am / pm
Woke up	____ am / pm
Total Hours slept	______
# of Disruptions	______

Symptoms	Relief Attempts	Results Notes

Activity

- ☐ Walk - distance ______
- ☐ Physiotherapy
- ☐ Light Exercise
- ☐ Gym
- ☐ Housework
- ☐ ______
- ☐ ______

Medications taken

- ☐ Diabetes
- ☐ Blood Pressure
- ☐ Pain Management (Prescription)
- ☐ Pain (overcounter): ______
- ☐ Natural Therapies: ______
- ☐ Other: ______
- ☐ Other: ______

Medications

- ☐ No Change
- ☐ Dosage Changed
- ☐ from ______
- ☐ to ______
- ☐ Medication Changed
- from ______
- to ______

DAY

Today,'s Dietary Intake

Drinks & Beverages

- ☐ Milk ☐ Juice ☐ Water
- ☐ Tea ☐ Coffee ☐ Soft / Energy Drink

Hydration

Breakfast	
	Blood Sugar: ______
	Blood Pressure: ______
	Temperature: ______
	Other: ______

Lunch	
	Blood Sugar: ______
	Blood Pressure: ______
	Temperature: ______
	Other: ______

Dinner	
	Blood Sugar: ______
	Blood Pressure: ______
	Temperature: ______
	Other: ______

Snacks	
	Blood Sugar: ______
	Blood Pressure: ______
	Temperature: ______
	Other: ______

- ☐ Fruit ☐ Vegetables ☐ Ginger Tea
- ☐ Grains & Cereals ☐ Fats

Daily Symptoms & Well-Being Tracker

DATE: ____ / ____ / ____

Today's Ratings

Pain	______ / 10	Anxiety	______ / 10	Went to bed	____ am / pm
Fatigue	______ / 10	Depression	______ / 10	Fell Asleep	____ am / pm
Weakness	______ / 10	Stress	______ / 10	Woke up	____ am / pm
Stiffness	______ / 10	Anger	______ / 10	Total Hours slept	______
General Mood	______			# of Disruptions	______

(Sleep)

Symptoms	Relief Attempts	Results Notes

Activity

- ☐ Walk - distance ______
- ☐ Physiotherapy
- ☐ Light Exercise
- ☐ Gym
- ☐ Housework
- ☐ ______
- ☐ ______

Medications taken

- ☐ Diabetes
- ☐ Blood Pressure
- ☐ Pain Management (Prescription)
- ☐ Pain (overcounter): ______
- ☐ Natural Therapies: ______
- ☐ Other: ______
- ☐ Other: ______

Medications

- ☐ No Change
- ☐ Dosage Changed
- ☐ from ______
- ☐ to ______
- ☐ Medication Changed
  - from ______
  - to ______

Daily Symptoms Tracker

Today,'s Dietary Intake

DAY

Drinks & Beverages

- ☐ Milk ☐ Juice ☐ Water
- ☐ Tea ☐ Coffee ☐ Soft / Energy Drink

Hydration

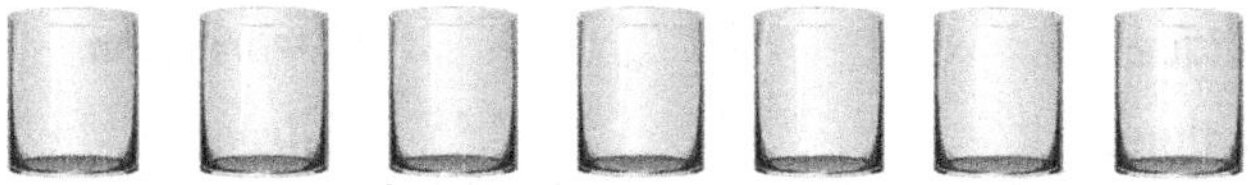

Breakfast	Blood Sugar:
	Blood Pressure:
	Temperature:
	Other:
Lunch	Blood Sugar:
	Blood Pressure:
	Temperature:
	Other:
Dinner	Blood Sugar:
	Blood Pressure:
	Temperature:
	Other:
Snacks	Blood Sugar:
	Blood Pressure:
	Temperature:
	Other:

- ☐ Fruit ☐ Vegetables ☐ Ginger Tea
- ☐ Grains & Cereals ☐ Fats

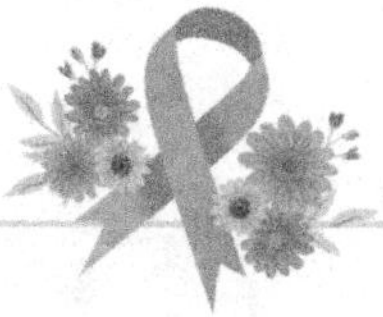

Daily Symptoms & Well-Being Tracker

DATE: ____ / ____ / ____

Today's Ratings

Pain	____ / 10	Anxiety	____ / 10
Fatigue	____ / 10	Depression	____ / 10
Weakness	____ / 10	Stress	____ / 10
Stiffness	____ / 10	Anger	____ / 10
General Mood	____		

Sleep

Went to bed	____ am / pm
Fell Asleep	____ am / pm
Woke up	____ am / pm
Total Hours slept	____
# of Disruptions	____

Symptoms	Relief Attempts	Results Notes

Activity

- ☐ Walk - distance ____
- ☐ Physiotherapy
- ☐ Light Exercise
- ☐ Gym
- ☐ Housework
- ☐ ____
- ☐ ____

Medications taken

- ☐ Diabetes
- ☐ Blood Pressure
- ☐ Pain Management (Prescription)
- ☐ Pain (overcounter): ____
- ☐ Natural Therapies: ____
- ☐ Other: ____
- ☐ Other: ____

Medications

- ☐ No Change
- ☐ Dosage Changed
- ☐ from ____
- ☐ to ____
- ☐ Medication Changed
  - from ____
  - to ____

DAY

Today,'s Dietary Intake

Drinks & Beverages

- ☐ Milk
- ☐ Juice
- ☐ Water
- ☐ Tea
- ☐ Coffee
- ☐ Soft / Energy Drink

Hydration

Breakfast	Blood Sugar: ______ Blood Pressure: ______ Temperature: ______ Other: ______
Lunch	Blood Sugar: ______ Blood Pressure: ______ Temperature: ______ Other: ______
Dinner	Blood Sugar: ______ Blood Pressure: ______ Temperature: ______ Other: ______
Snacks	Blood Sugar: ______ Blood Pressure: ______ Temperature: ______ Other: ______

- ☐ Fruit
- ☐ Vegetables
- ☐ Ginger Tea
- ☐ Grains & Cereals
- ☐ Fats

Daily Symptoms & Well-Being Tracker

DATE: ____ / ____ / ____

Today's Ratings

Pain	____ / 10	Anxiety	____ / 10		
Fatigue	____ / 10	Depression	____ / 10		
Weakness	____ / 10	Stress	____ / 10		
Stiffness	____ / 10	Anger	____ / 10		
General Mood	____				

Sleep

Went to bed	____ am / pm
Fell Asleep	____ am / pm
Woke up	____ am / pm
Total Hours slept	____
# of Disruptions	____

Symptoms	Relief Attempts	Results Notes

Activity

- ☐ Walk - distance ____
- ☐ Physiotherapy
- ☐ Light Exercise
- ☐ Gym
- ☐ Housework
- ☐ ____
- ☐ ____

Medications taken

- ☐ Diabetes
- ☐ Blood Pressure
- ☐ Pain Management (Prescription)
- ☐ Pain (overcounter): ____
- ☐ Natural Therapies: ____
- ☐ Other: ____
- ☐ Other: ____

Medications

- ☐ No Change
- ☐ Dosage Changed
- ☐ from ____
- ☐ to ____
- ☐ Medication Changed
  - from ____
  - to ____

DAY

Today,'s Dietary Intake

Drinks & Beverages

- ☐ Milk ☐ Juice ☐ Water
- ☐ Tea ☐ Coffee ☐ Soft / Energy Drink

Hydration

Breakfast

Blood Sugar: ______
Blood Pressure: ______
Temperature: ______
Other: ______

Lunch

Blood Sugar: ______
Blood Pressure: ______
Temperature: ______
Other: ______

Dinner

Blood Sugar: ______
Blood Pressure: ______
Temperature: ______
Other: ______

Snacks

Blood Sugar: ______
Blood Pressure: ______
Temperature: ______
Other: ______

- ☐ Fruit ☐ Vegetables ☐ Ginger Tea
- ☐ Grains & Cereals ☐ Fats

Daily Symptoms & Well-Being Tracker

DATE: ____ / ____ / ____

Today's Ratings

Pain	______ / 10	Anxiety	______ / 10		
Fatigue	______ / 10	Depression	______ / 10		
Weakness	______ / 10	Stress	______ / 10		
Stiffness	______ / 10	Anger	______ / 10		
General Mood	______				

Sleep

- Went to bed ______ am / pm
- Fell Asleep ______ am / pm
- Woke up ______ am / pm
- Total Hours slept ______
- # of Disruptions ______

Symptoms	Relief Attempts	Results Notes

Activity

- ☐ Walk - distance ______
- ☐ Physiotherapy
- ☐ Light Exercise
- ☐ Gym
- ☐ Housework
- ☐ ______
- ☐ ______

Medications taken

- ☐ Diabetes
- ☐ Blood Pressure
- ☐ Pain Management (Prescription)
- ☐ Pain (overcounter): ______
- ☐ Natural Therapies: ______
- ☐ Other: ______
- ☐ Other: ______

Medications

- ☐ No Change
- ☐ Dosage Changed
- ☐ from ______
- ☐ to ______
- ☐ Medication Changed
  - from ______
  - to ______

Today,'s Dietary Intake

DAY

Drinks & Beverages

- ☐ Milk ☐ Juice ☐ Water
- ☐ Tea ☐ Coffee ☐ Soft / Energy Drink

Hydration

Breakfast

Blood Sugar: ______
Blood Pressure: ______
Temperature: ______
Other: ______

Lunch

Blood Sugar: ______
Blood Pressure: ______
Temperature: ______
Other: ______

Dinner

Blood Sugar: ______
Blood Pressure: ______
Temperature: ______
Other: ______

Snacks

Blood Sugar: ______
Blood Pressure: ______
Temperature: ______
Other: ______

- ☐ Fruit ☐ Vegetables ☐ Ginger Tea
- ☐ Grains & Cereals ☐ Fats

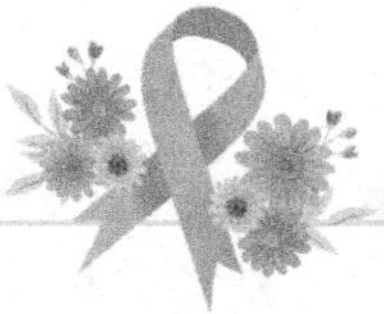

Weekly Summary

	Monday	Tuesday	Wednesday	Thursday	Friday	Saturday	Sunday
Pain							
Fatigue							
Weakness							
Stiffness							
Sleep (total Hours)							
# Disruptions							

Instructions:

Use the dots and dashes below to graph your ratings for the week - it helps to see things visually.

The bottom — equals 0; the middle — equals 5; and the top ◆ equals 10

Weekly Summary

	Monday	Tuesday	Wednesday	Thursday	Friday	Saturday	Sunday
Anxiety							
Depression							
Stress							
Anger							
Brain Fog / Forgetfulness							

Daily Symptoms & Well-Being Tracker

DATE: ____ / ____ / ____

Today's Ratings

Pain ________ / 10
Fatigue ________ / 10
Weakness ________ / 10
Stiffness ________ / 10
General Mood ________

Anxiety ________ / 10
Depression ________ / 10
Stress ________ / 10
Anger ________ / 10

Sleep

Went to bed ____ am / pm
Fell Asleep ____ am / pm
Woke up ____ am / pm
Total Hours slept ________
# of Disruptions ________

Symptoms	Relief Attempts	Results Notes

Activity

- ☐ Walk - distance ________
- ☐ Physiotherapy
- ☐ Light Exercise
- ☐ Gym
- ☐ Housework
- ☐ ________
- ☐ ________

Medications taken

- ☐ Diabetes
- ☐ Blood Pressure
- ☐ Pain Management (Prescription)
- ☐ Pain (overcounter): ________
- ☐ Natural Therapies: ________
- ☐ Other: ________
- ☐ Other: ________

Medications

- ☐ No Change
- ☐ Dosage Changed
- ☐ from ________
- ☐ to ________
- ☐ Medication Changed
  - from ________
  - to ________

Today,'s Dietary Intake

DAY

Drinks & Beverages

- ☐ Milk
- ☐ Juice
- ☐ Water
- ☐ Tea
- ☐ Coffee
- ☐ Soft / Energy Drink

Hydration

Breakfast

Blood Sugar: ______
Blood Pressure: ______
Temperature: ______
Other: ______

Lunch

Blood Sugar: ______
Blood Pressure: ______
Temperature: ______
Other: ______

Dinner

Blood Sugar: ______
Blood Pressure: ______
Temperature: ______
Other: ______

Snacks

Blood Sugar: ______
Blood Pressure: ______
Temperature: ______
Other: ______

- ☐ Fruit
- ☐ Vegetables
- ☐ Ginger Tea
- ☐ Grains & Cereals
- ☐ Fats

Daily Symptoms & Well-Being Tracker

DATE: ____ / ____ / ____

Today's Ratings

Pain ________ / 10
Fatigue ________ / 10
Weakness ________ / 10
Stiffness ________ / 10
General Mood ________

Anxiety ________ / 10
Depression ________ / 10
Stress ________ / 10
Anger ________ / 10

Sleep

Went to bed ____ am / pm
Fell Asleep ____ am / pm
Woke up ____ am / pm
Total Hours slept ________
# of Disruptions ________

Symptoms	Relief Attempts	Results Notes

Activity

- ☐ Walk - distance ________
- ☐ Physiotherapy
- ☐ Light Exercise
- ☐ Gym
- ☐ Housework
- ☐ ________
- ☐ ________

Medications taken

- ☐ Diabetes
- ☐ Blood Pressure
- ☐ Pain Management (Prescription)
- ☐ Pain (overcounter): ________
- ☐ Natural Therapies: ________
- ☐ Other: ________
- ☐ Other: ________

Medications

- ☐ No Change
- ☐ Dosage Changed
- ☐ from ________
- ☐ to ________
- ☐ Medication Changed
  - from ________
  - to ________

DAY

Today,'s Dietary Intake

Drinks & Beverages

- ☐ Milk ☐ Juice ☐ Water
- ☐ Tea ☐ Coffee ☐ Soft / Energy Drink

Hydration

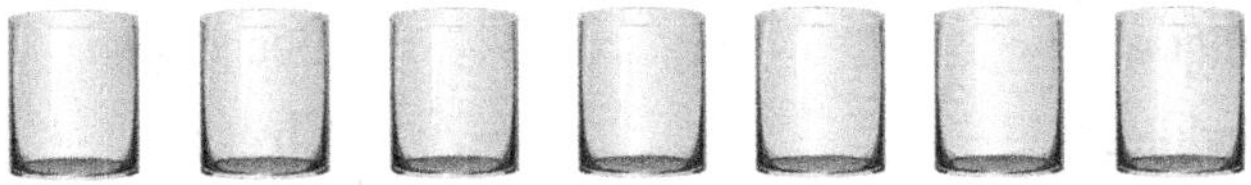

Breakfast

Blood Sugar: ______
Blood Pressure: ______
Temperature: ______
Other: ______

Lunch

Blood Sugar: ______
Blood Pressure: ______
Temperature: ______
Other: ______

Dinner

Blood Sugar: ______
Blood Pressure: ______
Temperature: ______
Other: ______

Snacks

Blood Sugar: ______
Blood Pressure: ______
Temperature: ______
Other: ______

- ☐ Fruit ☐ Vegetables ☐ Ginger Tea
- ☐ Grains & Cereals ☐ Fats

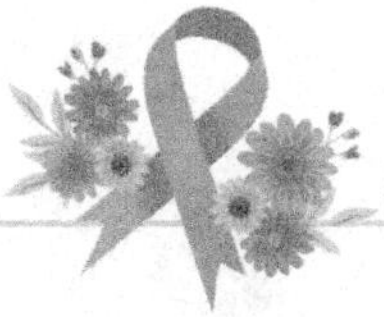

Daily Symptoms & Well-Being Tracker

DATE: ____ / ____ / ____

Today's Ratings

Pain ______ / 10	Anxiety ______ / 10	
Fatigue ______ / 10	Depression ______ / 10	
Weakness ______ / 10	Stress ______ / 10	
Stiffness ______ / 10	Anger ______ / 10	
General Mood ______		

Sleep

- Went to bed ____ am / pm
- Fell Asleep ____ am / pm
- Woke up ____ am / pm
- Total Hours slept ______
- # of Disruptions ______

Symptoms	Relief Attempts	Results Notes

Activity

- ☐ Walk - distance ______
- ☐ Physiotherapy
- ☐ Light Exercise
- ☐ Gym
- ☐ Housework
- ☐ ______
- ☐ ______

Medications taken

- ☐ Diabetes
- ☐ Blood Pressure
- ☐ Pain Management (Prescription)
- ☐ Pain (overcounter): ______
- ☐ Natural Therapies: ______
- ☐ Other: ______
- ☐ Other: ______

Medications

- ☐ No Change
- ☐ Dosage Changed
- ☐ from ______
- ☐ to ______
- ☐ Medication Changed
  - from ______
  - to ______

DAY

Today,'s Dietary Intake

Drinks & Beverages

- ☐ Milk
- ☐ Juice
- ☐ Water
- ☐ Tea
- ☐ Coffee
- ☐ Soft / Energy Drink

Hydration

Breakfast

Blood Sugar: ______
Blood Pressure: ______
Temperature: ______
Other: ______

Lunch

Blood Sugar: ______
Blood Pressure: ______
Temperature: ______
Other: ______

Dinner

Blood Sugar: ______
Blood Pressure: ______
Temperature: ______
Other: ______

Snacks

Blood Sugar: ______
Blood Pressure: ______
Temperature: ______
Other: ______

- ☐ Fruit
- ☐ Vegetables
- ☐ Ginger Tea
- ☐ Grains & Cereals
- ☐ Fats

Daily Symptoms & Well-Being Tracker

DATE: ____ / ____ / ____

Today's Ratings

Pain	______ / 10	Anxiety	______ / 10	Went to bed	____ am / pm
Fatigue	______ / 10	Depression	______ / 10	Fell Asleep	____ am / pm
Weakness	______ / 10	Stress	______ / 10	Woke up	____ am / pm
Stiffness	______ / 10	Anger	______ / 10	Total Hours slept	______
General Mood	______			# of Disruptions	______

Sleep

Symptoms	Relief Attempts	Results Notes

Activity

- ☐ Walk - distance ______
- ☐ Physiotherapy
- ☐ Light Exercise
- ☐ Gym
- ☐ Housework
- ☐ ______
- ☐ ______

Medications taken

- ☐ Diabetes
- ☐ Blood Pressure
- ☐ Pain Management (Prescription)
- ☐ Pain (overcounter): ______
- ☐ Natural Therapies: ______
- ☐ Other: ______
- ☐ Other: ______

Medications

- ☐ No Change
- ☐ Dosage Changed
- ☐ from ______
- ☐ to ______
- ☐ Medication Changed
- from ______
- to ______

Daily Symptoms Tracker

Today,'s Dietary Intake

DAY

Drinks & Beverages

- ☐ Milk
- ☐ Juice
- ☐ Water
- ☐ Tea
- ☐ Coffee
- ☐ Soft / Energy Drink

Hydration

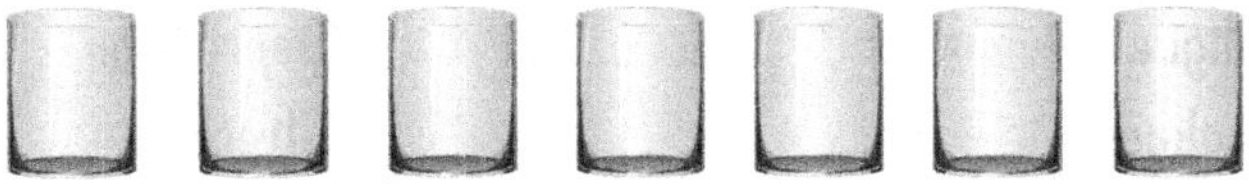

Breakfast

Blood Sugar: ______
Blood Pressure: ______
Temperature: ______
Other: ______

Lunch

Blood Sugar: ______
Blood Pressure: ______
Temperature: ______
Other: ______

Dinner

Blood Sugar: ______
Blood Pressure: ______
Temperature: ______
Other: ______

Snacks

Blood Sugar: ______
Blood Pressure: ______
Temperature: ______
Other: ______

- ☐ Fruit
- ☐ Vegetables
- ☐ Ginger Tea
- ☐ Grains & Cereals
- ☐ Fats

Daily Symptoms & Well-Being Tracker

DATE: ____ / ____ / ____

Today's Ratings

Pain ________ / 10
Fatigue ________ / 10
Weakness ________ / 10
Stiffness ________ / 10
General Mood ________

Anxiety ________ / 10
Depression ________ / 10
Stress ________ / 10
Anger ________ / 10

Sleep

Went to bed ____ am / pm
Fell Asleep ____ am / pm
Woke up ____ am / pm
Total Hours slept ________
# of Disruptions ________

Symptoms	Relief Attempts	Results Notes

Activity

- ☐ Walk - distance ________
- ☐ Physiotherapy
- ☐ Light Exercise
- ☐ Gym
- ☐ Housework
- ☐ ________
- ☐ ________

Medications taken

- ☐ Diabetes
- ☐ Blood Pressure
- ☐ Pain Management (Prescription)
- ☐ Pain (overcounter): ________
- ☐ Natural Therapies: ________
- ☐ Other: ________
- ☐ Other: ________

Medications

- ☐ No Change
- ☐ Dosage Changed
- ☐ from ________
- ☐ to ________
- ☐ Medication Changed
  - from ________
  - to ________

Daily Symptoms Tracker

Today,'s Dietary Intake

DAY

Drinks & Beverages

☐ Milk ☐ Juice ☐ Water
☐ Tea ☐ Coffee ☐ Soft / Energy Drink

Hydration

☐ ☐ ☐ ☐ ☐ ☐ ☐

Breakfast

Blood Sugar: ______
Blood Pressure: ______
Temperature: ______
Other: ______

Lunch

Blood Sugar: ______
Blood Pressure: ______
Temperature: ______
Other: ______

Dinner

Blood Sugar: ______
Blood Pressure: ______
Temperature: ______
Other: ______

Snacks

Blood Sugar: ______
Blood Pressure: ______
Temperature: ______
Other: ______

☐ Fruit ☐ Vegetables ☐ Ginger Tea
☐ Grains & Cereals ☐ Fats

Daily Symptoms & Well-Being Tracker

DATE: ____ / ____ / ____

Today's Ratings

Pain	______ / 10
Fatigue	______ / 10
Weakness	______ / 10
Stiffness	______ / 10
General Mood	______
Anxiety	______ / 10
Depression	______ / 10
Stress	______ / 10
Anger	______ / 10

Sleep

Went to bed	____ am / pm
Fell Asleep	____ am / pm
Woke up	____ am / pm
Total Hours slept	______
# of Disruptions	______

Symptoms	Relief Attempts	Results Notes

Activity

- ☐ Walk - distance ______
- ☐ Physiotherapy
- ☐ Light Exercise
- ☐ Gym
- ☐ Housework
- ☐ ______
- ☐ ______

Medications taken

- ☐ Diabetes
- ☐ Blood Pressure
- ☐ Pain Management (Prescription)
- ☐ Pain (overcounter): ______
- ☐ Natural Therapies: ______
- ☐ Other: ______
- ☐ Other: ______

Medications

- ☐ No Change
- ☐ Dosage Changed
- ☐ from ______
- ☐ to ______
- ☐ Medication Changed
  - from ______
  - to ______

Today,'s Dietary Intake

DAY

Drinks & Beverages

- ☐ Milk ☐ Juice ☐ Water
- ☐ Tea ☐ Coffee ☐ Soft / Energy Drink

Hydration

Breakfast

Blood Sugar: ______

Blood Pressure: ______

Temperature: ______

Other: ______

Lunch

Blood Sugar: ______

Blood Pressure: ______

Temperature: ______

Other: ______

Dinner

Blood Sugar: ______

Blood Pressure: ______

Temperature: ______

Other: ______

Snacks

Blood Sugar: ______

Blood Pressure: ______

Temperature: ______

Other: ______

- ☐ Fruit ☐ Vegetables ☐ Ginger Tea
- ☐ Grains & Cereals ☐ Fats

Daily Symptoms & Well-Being Tracker

DATE: ____ / ____ / ____

Today's Ratings

Pain ________ / 10
Fatigue ________ / 10
Weakness ________ / 10
Stiffness ________ / 10
General Mood ________

Anxiety ________ / 10
Depression ________ / 10
Stress ________ / 10
Anger ________ / 10

Sleep

Went to bed ______ am / pm
Fell Asleep ______ am / pm
Woke up ______ am / pm
Total Hours slept ________
# of Disruptions ________

Symptoms	Relief Attempts	Results Notes

Activity

- ☐ Walk - distance ________
- ☐ Physiotherapy
- ☐ Light Exercise
- ☐ Gym
- ☐ Housework
- ☐ ________
- ☐ ________

Medications taken

- ☐ Diabetes
- ☐ Blood Pressure
- ☐ Pain Management (Prescription)
- ☐ Pain (overcounter): ________
- ☐ Natural Therapies: ________
- ☐ Other: ________
- ☐ Other: ________

Medications

- ☐ No Change
- ☐ Dosage Changed
- ☐ from ________
- ☐ to ________
- ☐ Medication Changed
  - from ________
  - to ________

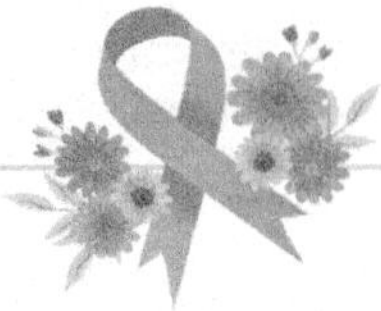

DAY

Today,'s Dietary Intake

Drinks & Beverages

- ☐ Milk
- ☐ Juice
- ☐ Water
- ☐ Tea
- ☐ Coffee
- ☐ Soft / Energy Drink

Hydration

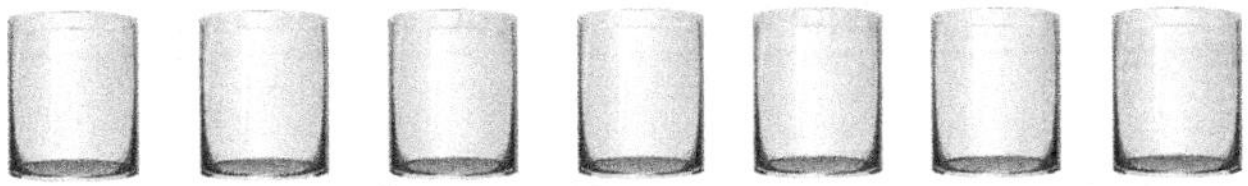

Breakfast	
	Blood Sugar:
	Blood Pressure:
	Temperature:
	Other:

Lunch	
	Blood Sugar:
	Blood Pressure:
	Temperature:
	Other:

Dinner	
	Blood Sugar:
	Blood Pressure:
	Temperature:
	Other:

Snacks	
	Blood Sugar:
	Blood Pressure:
	Temperature:
	Other:

- ☐ Fruit
- ☐ Vegetables
- ☐ Ginger Tea
- ☐ Grains & Cereals
- ☐ Fats

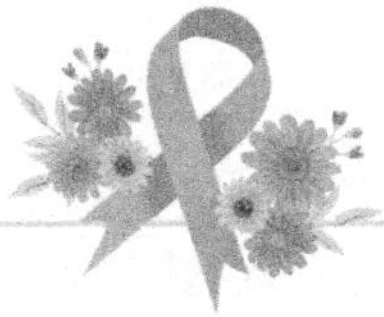

Weekly Summary

	Monday	Tuesday	Wednesday	Thursday	Friday	Saturday	Sunday
Pain							
Fatigue							
Weakness							
Stiffness							
Sleep (total Hours)	______	______	______	______	______	______	______
# Disruptions	______	______	______	______	______	______	______

Instructions:

Use the dots and dashes below to graph your ratings for the week – it helps to see things visually.

The bottom -- equals 0; the middle -- equals 5; and the top ◆ equals 10

Weekly Summary

	Monday	Tuesday	Wednesday	Thursday	Friday	Saturday	Sunday
Anxiety							
Depression							
Stress							
Anger							
Brain Fog / Forgetfulness							

Daily Symptoms & Well-Being Tracker

DATE: ____ / ____ / ____

Today's Ratings

Pain	______ / 10	Anxiety	______ / 10
Fatigue	______ / 10	Depression	______ / 10
Weakness	______ / 10	Stress	______ / 10
Stiffness	______ / 10	Anger	______ / 10
General Mood	______		

Sleep

Went to bed	____ am / pm
Fell Asleep	____ am / pm
Woke up	____ am / pm
Total Hours slept	______
# of Disruptions	______

Symptoms	Relief Attempts	Results Notes

Activity

- ☐ Walk - distance ______
- ☐ Physiotherapy
- ☐ Light Exercise
- ☐ Gym
- ☐ Housework
- ☐ ______
- ☐ ______

Medications taken

- ☐ Diabetes
- ☐ Blood Pressure
- ☐ Pain Management (Prescription)
- ☐ Pain (overcounter): ______
- ☐ Natural Therapies: ______
- ☐ Other: ______
- ☐ Other: ______

Medications

- ☐ No Change
- ☐ Dosage Changed
- ☐ from ______
- ☐ to ______
- ☐ Medication Changed
  - from ______
  - to ______

Today,'s Dietary Intake

DAY

Drinks & Beverages

- ☐ Milk ☐ Juice ☐ Water
- ☐ Tea ☐ Coffee ☐ Soft / Energy Drink

Hydration

Breakfast

Blood Sugar: ______
Blood Pressure: ______
Temperature: ______
Other: ______

Lunch

Blood Sugar: ______
Blood Pressure: ______
Temperature: ______
Other: ______

Dinner

Blood Sugar: ______
Blood Pressure: ______
Temperature: ______
Other: ______

Snacks

Blood Sugar: ______
Blood Pressure: ______
Temperature: ______
Other: ______

- ☐ Fruit ☐ Vegetables ☐ Ginger Tea
- ☐ Grains & Cereals ☐ Fats

Daily Symptoms & Well-Being Tracker

DATE: ____ / ____ / ____

Today's Ratings

Pain	______ / 10
Fatigue	______ / 10
Weakness	______ / 10
Stiffness	______ / 10
General Mood	______

Anxiety	______ / 10
Depression	______ / 10
Stress	______ / 10
Anger	______ / 10

Sleep

Went to bed	____ am / pm
Fell Asleep	____ am / pm
Woke up	____ am / pm
Total Hours slept	______
# of Disruptions	______

Symptoms	Relief Attempts	Results Notes

Activity

- ☐ Walk - distance ______
- ☐ Physiotherapy
- ☐ Light Exercise
- ☐ Gym
- ☐ Housework
- ☐ ______
- ☐ ______

Medications taken

- ☐ Diabetes
- ☐ Blood Pressure
- ☐ Pain Management (Prescription)
- ☐ Pain (overcounter): ______
- ☐ Natural Therapies: ______
- ☐ Other: ______
- ☐ Other: ______

Medications

- ☐ No Change
- ☐ Dosage Changed
- ☐ from ______
- ☐ to ______
- ☐ Medication Changed
- from ______
- to ______

DAY

Today,'s Dietary Intake

Drinks & Beverages

☐ Milk ☐ Juice ☐ Water

☐ Tea ☐ Coffee ☐ Soft / Energy Drink

Hydration

Breakfast

Blood Sugar: ____________

Blood Pressure: ____________

Temperature: ____________

Other: ____________

Lunch

Blood Sugar: ____________

Blood Pressure: ____________

Temperature: ____________

Other: ____________

Dinner

Blood Sugar: ____________

Blood Pressure: ____________

Temperature: ____________

Other: ____________

Snacks

Blood Sugar: ____________

Blood Pressure: ____________

Temperature: ____________

Other: ____________

☐ Fruit ☐ Vegetables ☐ Ginger Tea

☐ Grains & Cereals ☐ Fats

Daily Symptoms & Well-Being Tracker

DATE: ____ / ____ / ____

Today's Ratings

Pain	______ / 10	Anxiety	______ / 10
Fatigue	______ / 10	Depression	______ / 10
Weakness	______ / 10	Stress	______ / 10
Stiffness	______ / 10	Anger	______ / 10
General Mood	______		

Sleep

Went to bed	____ am / pm
Fell Asleep	____ am / pm
Woke up	____ am / pm
Total Hours slept	______
# of Disruptions	______

Symptoms	Relief Attempts	Results Notes

Activity

- ☐ Walk - distance ______
- ☐ Physiotherapy
- ☐ Light Exercise
- ☐ Gym
- ☐ Housework
- ☐ ______
- ☐ ______

Medications taken

- ☐ Diabetes
- ☐ Blood Pressure
- ☐ Pain Management (Prescription)
- ☐ Pain (overcounter): ______
- ☐ Natural Therapies: ______
- ☐ Other: ______
- ☐ Other: ______

Medications

- ☐ No Change
- ☐ Dosage Changed
- ☐ from ______
- ☐ to ______
- ☐ Medication Changed
  - from ______
  - to ______

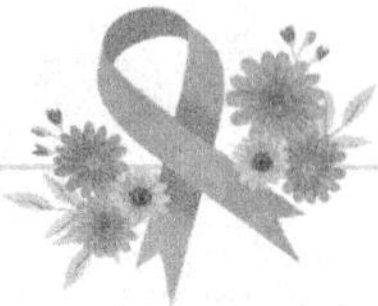

Daily Symptoms Tracker

Today,'s Dietary Intake

DAY

Drinks & Beverages

- ☐ Milk
- ☐ Juice
- ☐ Water
- ☐ Tea
- ☐ Coffee
- ☐ Soft / Energy Drink

Hydration

Breakfast

Blood Sugar: ____________

Blood Pressure: ____________

Temperature: ____________

Other: ____________

Lunch

Blood Sugar: ____________

Blood Pressure: ____________

Temperature: ____________

Other: ____________

Dinner

Blood Sugar: ____________

Blood Pressure: ____________

Temperature: ____________

Other: ____________

Snacks

Blood Sugar: ____________

Blood Pressure: ____________

Temperature: ____________

Other: ____________

- ☐ Fruit
- ☐ Vegetables
- ☐ Ginger Tea
- ☐ Grains & Cereals
- ☐ Fats

Daily Symptoms & Well-Being Tracker

DATE: ____ / ____ / ____

Today's Ratings

Pain	______ / 10	Anxiety	______ / 10		
Fatigue	______ / 10	Depression	______ / 10		
Weakness	______ / 10	Stress	______ / 10		
Stiffness	______ / 10	Anger	______ / 10		
General Mood	______				

Sleep

- Went to bed ____ am / pm
- Fell Asleep ____ am / pm
- Woke up ____ am / pm
- Total Hours slept ______
- # of Disruptions ______

Symptoms	Relief Attempts	Results Notes

Activity

- ☐ Walk - distance ______
- ☐ Physiotherapy
- ☐ Light Exercise
- ☐ Gym
- ☐ Housework
- ☐ ______
- ☐ ______

Medications taken

- ☐ Diabetes
- ☐ Blood Pressure
- ☐ Pain Management (Prescription)
- ☐ Pain (overcounter): ______
- ☐ Natural Therapies: ______
- ☐ Other: ______
- ☐ Other: ______

Medications

- ☐ No Change
- ☐ Dosage Changed
- ☐ from ______
- ☐ to ______
- ☐ Medication Changed
- from ______
- to ______

DAY

Today,'s Dietary Intake

Drinks & Beverages

- ☐ Milk ☐ Juice ☐ Water
- ☐ Tea ☐ Coffee ☐ Soft / Energy Drink

Hydration

Breakfast

Blood Sugar: ____________
Blood Pressure: ____________
Temperature: ____________
Other: ____________

Lunch

Blood Sugar: ____________
Blood Pressure: ____________
Temperature: ____________
Other: ____________

Dinner

Blood Sugar: ____________
Blood Pressure: ____________
Temperature: ____________
Other: ____________

Snacks

Blood Sugar: ____________
Blood Pressure: ____________
Temperature: ____________
Other: ____________

- ☐ Fruit ☐ Vegetables ☐ Ginger Tea
- ☐ Grains & Cereals ☐ Fats

Daily Symptoms & Well-Being Tracker

DATE: ____ / ____ / ____

Today's Ratings

Pain	______ / 10	Anxiety	______ / 10
Fatigue	______ / 10	Depression	______ / 10
Weakness	______ / 10	Stress	______ / 10
Stiffness	______ / 10	Anger	______ / 10
General Mood	______		

Sleep

Went to bed	____ am / pm
Fell Asleep	____ am / pm
Woke up	____ am / pm
Total Hours slept	______
# of Disruptions	______

Symptoms	Relief Attempts	Results Notes

Activity

- ☐ Walk - distance ______
- ☐ Physiotherapy
- ☐ Light Exercise
- ☐ Gym
- ☐ Housework
- ☐ ______
- ☐ ______

Medications taken

- ☐ Diabetes
- ☐ Blood Pressure
- ☐ Pain Management (Prescription)
- ☐ Pain (overcounter): ______
- ☐ Natural Therapies: ______
- ☐ Other: ______
- ☐ Other: ______

Medications

- ☐ No Change
- ☐ Dosage Changed
- ☐ from ______
- ☐ to ______
- ☐ Medication Changed
  - from ______
  - to ______

Today,'s Dietary Intake

DAY

Drinks & Beverages

☐ Milk ☐ Juice ☐ Water
☐ Tea ☐ Coffee ☐ Soft / Energy Drink

Hydration

Breakfast	Blood Sugar: ____
____	Blood Pressure: ____
____	Temperature: ____
____	Other: ____
Lunch	
____	Blood Sugar: ____
____	Blood Pressure: ____
____	Temperature: ____
____	Other: ____
Dinner	
____	Blood Sugar: ____
____	Blood Pressure: ____
____	Temperature: ____
____	Other: ____
____	
Snacks	
____	Blood Sugar: ____
____	Blood Pressure: ____
____	Temperature: ____
____	Other: ____

☐ Fruit ☐ Vegetables ☐ Ginger Tea
☐ Grains & Cereals ☐ Fats

Daily Symptoms & Well-Being Tracker

DATE: ____ / ____ / ____

Today's Ratings

Pain	____ / 10	Anxiety	____ / 10	Went to bed	____ am / pm
Fatigue	____ / 10	Depression	____ / 10	Fell Asleep	____ am / pm
Weakness	____ / 10	Stress	____ / 10	Woke up	____ am / pm
Stiffness	____ / 10	Anger	____ / 10	Total Hours slept	____
General Mood	____			# of Disruptions	____

Sleep

Symptoms	Relief Attempts	Results Notes

Activity

- ☐ Walk - distance ____
- ☐ Physiotherapy
- ☐ Light Exercise
- ☐ Gym
- ☐ Housework
- ☐ ____
- ☐ ____

Medications taken

- ☐ Diabetes
- ☐ Blood Pressure
- ☐ Pain Management (Prescription)
- ☐ Pain (overcounter): ____
- ☐ Natural Therapies: ____
- ☐ Other: ____
- ☐ Other: ____

Medications

- ☐ No Change
- ☐ Dosage Changed
- ☐ from ____
- ☐ to ____
- ☐ Medication Changed
  - from ____
  - to ____

DAY

Today,'s Dietary Intake

Drinks & Beverages

- ☐ Milk ☐ Juice ☐ Water
- ☐ Tea ☐ Coffee ☐ Soft / Energy Drink

Hydration

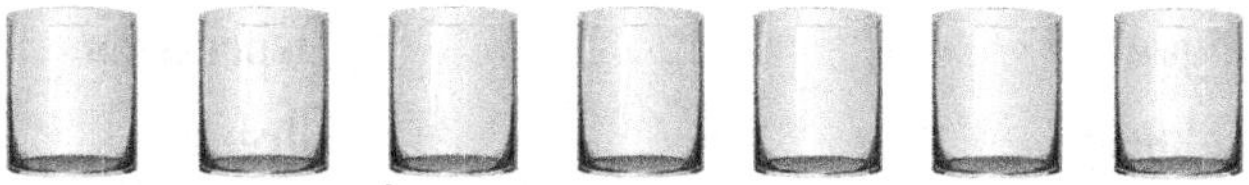

Breakfast

Blood Sugar: ______
Blood Pressure: ______
Temperature: ______
Other: ______

Lunch

Blood Sugar: ______
Blood Pressure: ______
Temperature: ______
Other: ______

Dinner

Blood Sugar: ______
Blood Pressure: ______
Temperature: ______
Other: ______

Snacks

Blood Sugar: ______
Blood Pressure: ______
Temperature: ______
Other: ______

- ☐ Fruit ☐ Vegetables ☐ Ginger Tea
- ☐ Grains & Cereals ☐ Fats

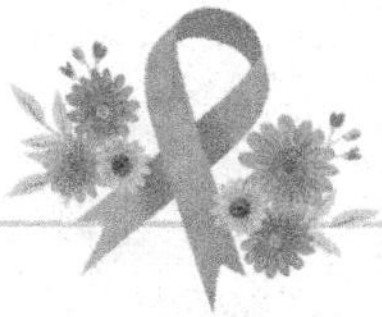

Daily Symptoms & Well-Being Tracker

DATE: ____ / ____ / ____

Today's Ratings

Pain	______ / 10	Anxiety	______ / 10		
Fatigue	______ / 10	Depression	______ / 10		
Weakness	______ / 10	Stress	______ / 10		
Stiffness	______ / 10	Anger	______ / 10		
General Mood	______				

Sleep

Went to bed ____ am / pm
Fell Asleep ____ am / pm
Woke up ____ am / pm
Total Hours slept ______
# of Disruptions ______

Symptoms	Relief Attempts	Results Notes

Activity

- ☐ Walk - distance ______
- ☐ Physiotherapy
- ☐ Light Exercise
- ☐ Gym
- ☐ Housework
- ☐ ______
- ☐ ______

Medications taken

- ☐ Diabetes
- ☐ Blood Pressure
- ☐ Pain Management (Prescription)
- ☐ Pain (overcounter): ______
- ☐ Natural Therapies: ______
- ☐ Other: ______
- ☐ Other: ______

Medications

- ☐ No Change
- ☐ Dosage Changed
- ☐ from ______
- ☐ to ______
- ☐ Medication Changed
  - from ______
  - to ______

Today,'s Dietary Intake

DAY

Drinks & Beverages

☐ Milk ☐ Juice ☐ Water

☐ Tea ☐ Coffee ☐ Soft / Energy Drink

Hydration

Breakfast

Blood Sugar: ______
Blood Pressure: ______
Temperature: ______
Other: ______

Lunch

Blood Sugar: ______
Blood Pressure: ______
Temperature: ______
Other: ______

Dinner

Blood Sugar: ______
Blood Pressure: ______
Temperature: ______
Other: ______

Snacks

Blood Sugar: ______
Blood Pressure: ______
Temperature: ______
Other: ______

☐ Fruit ☐ Vegetables ☐ Ginger Tea

☐ Grains & Cereals ☐ Fats

Weekly Summary

	Monday	Tuesday	Wednesday	Thursday	Friday	Saturday	Sunday
Pain							
Fatigue							
Weakness							
Stiffness							
Sleep (total Hours)							
# Disruptions							

Instructions:

Use the dots and dashes below to graph your ratings for the week – it helps to see things visually.

The bottom -- equals 0; the middle -- equals 5; and the top ◆ equals 10

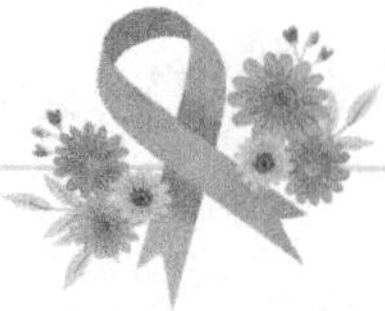

Weekly Summary

	Monday	Tuesday	Wednesday	Thursday	Friday	Saturday	Sunday
Anxiety							
Depression							
Stress							
Anger							
Brain Fog / Forgetfulness							

Daily Symptoms & Well-Being Tracker

DATE: ____ / ____ / ____

Today's Ratings

Pain ________ / 10
Fatigue ________ / 10
Weakness ________ / 10
Stiffness ________ / 10
General Mood ________

Anxiety ________ / 10
Depression ________ / 10
Stress ________ / 10
Anger ________ / 10

Sleep

Went to bed ______ am / pm
Fell Asleep ______ am / pm
Woke up ______ am / pm
Total Hours slept ________
# of Disruptions ________

Symptoms	Relief Attempts	Results Notes

Activity

- ☐ Walk - distance ________
- ☐ Physiotherapy
- ☐ Light Exercise
- ☐ Gym
- ☐ Housework
- ☐ ________
- ☐ ________

Medications taken

- ☐ Diabetes
- ☐ Blood Pressure
- ☐ Pain Management (Prescription)
- ☐ Pain (overcounter): ________
- ☐ Natural Therapies: ________
- ☐ Other: ________
- ☐ Other: ________

Medications

- ☐ No Change
- ☐ Dosage Changed
- ☐ from ________
- ☐ to ________
- ☐ Medication Changed
  - from ________
  - to ________

Daily Symptoms Tracker

Today.'s Dietary Intake

DAY

Drinks & Beverages

- [ ] Milk
- [ ] Juice
- [ ] Water
- [ ] Tea
- [ ] Coffee
- [ ] Soft / Energy Drink

Hydration

Breakfast

Blood Sugar: ____________
Blood Pressure: ____________
Temperature: ____________
Other: ____________

Lunch

Blood Sugar: ____________
Blood Pressure: ____________
Temperature: ____________
Other: ____________

Dinner

Blood Sugar: ____________
Blood Pressure: ____________
Temperature: ____________
Other: ____________

Snacks

Blood Sugar: ____________
Blood Pressure: ____________
Temperature: ____________
Other: ____________

- [ ] Fruit
- [ ] Vegetables
- [ ] Ginger Tea
- [ ] Grains & Cereals
- [ ] Fats

Daily Symptoms & Well-Being Tracker

DATE: ____ / ____ / ____

Today's Ratings

Pain	______ / 10	Anxiety	______ / 10
Fatigue	______ / 10	Depression	______ / 10
Weakness	______ / 10	Stress	______ / 10
Stiffness	______ / 10	Anger	______ / 10
General Mood	______		

Sleep

Went to bed ____ am / pm

Fell Asleep ____ am / pm

Woke up ____ am / pm

Total Hours slept ______

# of Disruptions ______

Symptoms	Relief Attempts	Results Notes

Activity

- ☐ Walk - distance ______
- ☐ Physiotherapy
- ☐ Light Exercise
- ☐ Gym
- ☐ Housework
- ☐ ______
- ☐ ______

Medications taken

- ☐ Diabetes
- ☐ Blood Pressure
- ☐ Pain Management (Prescription)
- ☐ Pain (overcounter): ______
- ☐ Natural Therapies: ______
- ☐ Other: ______
- ☐ Other: ______

Medications

- ☐ No Change
- ☐ Dosage Changed
- ☐ from ______
- ☐ to ______
- ☐ Medication Changed
  - from ______
  - to ______

Today,'s Dietary Intake

DAY

Drinks & Beverages

- ☐ Milk ☐ Juice ☐ Water
- ☐ Tea ☐ Coffee ☐ Soft / Energy Drink

Hydration

Breakfast

Blood Sugar: ______
Blood Pressure: ______
Temperature: ______
Other: ______

Lunch

Blood Sugar: ______
Blood Pressure: ______
Temperature: ______
Other: ______

Dinner

Blood Sugar: ______
Blood Pressure: ______
Temperature: ______
Other: ______

Snacks

Blood Sugar: ______
Blood Pressure: ______
Temperature: ______
Other: ______

- ☐ Fruit ☐ Vegetables ☐ Ginger Tea
- ☐ Grains & Cereals ☐ Fats

Daily Symptoms & Well-Being Tracker

DATE: ____ / ____ / ____

Today's Ratings

Pain	______ / 10	Anxiety	______ / 10	Went to bed	____ am / pm
Fatigue	______ / 10	Depression	______ / 10	Fell Asleep	____ am / pm
Weakness	______ / 10	Stress	______ / 10	Woke up	____ am / pm
Stiffness	______ / 10	Anger	______ / 10	Total Hours slept	________
General Mood	________			# of Disruptions	________

(The third column is headed "Sleep".)

Symptoms	Relief Attempts	Results Notes

Activity

- ☐ Walk - distance ________
- ☐ Physiotherapy
- ☐ Light Exercise
- ☐ Gym
- ☐ Housework
- ☐ ________
- ☐ ________

Medications taken

- ☐ Diabetes
- ☐ Blood Pressure
- ☐ Pain Management (Prescription)
- ☐ Pain (overcounter): ________
- ☐ Natural Therapies: ________
- ☐ Other: ________
- ☐ Other: ________

Medications

- ☐ No Change
- ☐ Dosage Changed
- ☐ from ________
- ☐ to ________
- ☐ Medication Changed
  - from ________
  - to ________

Daily Symptoms Tracker

Today.'s Dietary Intake

DAY

Drinks & Beverages

- ☐ Milk
- ☐ Juice
- ☐ Water
- ☐ Tea
- ☐ Coffee
- ☐ Soft / Energy Drink

Hydration

Breakfast

Blood Sugar: ____________

Blood Pressure: ____________

Temperature: ____________

Other: ____________

Lunch

Blood Sugar: ____________

Blood Pressure: ____________

Temperature: ____________

Other: ____________

Dinner

Blood Sugar: ____________

Blood Pressure: ____________

Temperature: ____________

Other: ____________

Snacks

Blood Sugar: ____________

Blood Pressure: ____________

Temperature: ____________

Other: ____________

- ☐ Fruit
- ☐ Vegetables
- ☐ Ginger Tea
- ☐ Grains & Cereals
- ☐ Fats

Daily Symptoms & Well-Being Tracker

DATE: ____ / ____ / ____

Today's Ratings

Pain	____ / 10	Anxiety	____ / 10
Fatigue	____ / 10	Depression	____ / 10
Weakness	____ / 10	Stress	____ / 10
Stiffness	____ / 10	Anger	____ / 10
General Mood	____		

Sleep

Went to bed	____ am / pm
Fell Asleep	____ am / pm
Woke up	____ am / pm
Total Hours slept	____
# of Disruptions	____

Symptoms	Relief Attempts	Results Notes

Activity

- ☐ Walk - distance ____
- ☐ Physiotherapy
- ☐ Light Exercise
- ☐ Gym
- ☐ Housework
- ☐ ____
- ☐ ____

Medications taken

- ☐ Diabetes
- ☐ Blood Pressure
- ☐ Pain Management (Prescription)
- ☐ Pain (overcounter): ____
- ☐ Natural Therapies: ____
- ☐ Other: ____
- ☐ Other: ____

Medications

- ☐ No Change
- ☐ Dosage Changed
- ☐ from ____
- ☐ to ____
- ☐ Medication Changed
  - from ____
  - to ____

DAY

Today,'s Dietary Intake

Drinks & Beverages

- ☐ Milk ☐ Juice ☐ Water
- ☐ Tea ☐ Coffee ☐ Soft / Energy Drink

Hydration

Breakfast

____

____

____

Blood Sugar: ______

Blood Pressure: ______

Temperature: ______

Other: ______

Lunch

____

____

____

____

Blood Sugar: ______

Blood Pressure: ______

Temperature: ______

Other: ______

Dinner

____

____

____

____

____

Blood Sugar: ______

Blood Pressure: ______

Temperature: ______

Other: ______

Snacks

____

____

____

____

Blood Sugar: ______

Blood Pressure: ______

Temperature: ______

Other: ______

- ☐ Fruit ☐ Vegetables ☐ Ginger Tea
- ☐ Grains & Cereals ☐ Fats

Daily Symptoms & Well-Being Tracker

DATE: ____ / ____ / ____

Today's Ratings

Pain	______ / 10	Anxiety	______ / 10	Went to bed	____ am / pm
Fatigue	______ / 10	Depression	______ / 10	Fell Asleep	____ am / pm
Weakness	______ / 10	Stress	______ / 10	Woke up	____ am / pm
Stiffness	______ / 10	Anger	______ / 10	Total Hours slept	______
General Mood	______			# of Disruptions	______

(Sleep)

Symptoms	Relief Attempts	Results Notes

Activity

- ☐ Walk - distance ______
- ☐ Physiotherapy
- ☐ Light Exercise
- ☐ Gym
- ☐ Housework
- ☐ ______
- ☐ ______

Medications taken

- ☐ Diabetes
- ☐ Blood Pressure
- ☐ Pain Management (Prescription)
- ☐ Pain (overcounter): ______
- ☐ Natural Therapies: ______
- ☐ Other: ______
- ☐ Other: ______

Medications

- ☐ No Change
- ☐ Dosage Changed
- ☐ from ______
- ☐ to ______
- ☐ Medication Changed
- from ______
- to ______

DAY

Today,'s Dietary Intake

Drinks & Beverages

- ☐ Milk ☐ Juice ☐ Water
- ☐ Tea ☐ Coffee ☐ Soft / Energy Drink

Hydration

☐ ☐ ☐ ☐ ☐ ☐ ☐

Breakfast	Blood Sugar: ______ Blood Pressure: ______ Temperature: ______ Other: ______
Lunch	Blood Sugar: ______ Blood Pressure: ______ Temperature: ______ Other: ______
Dinner	Blood Sugar: ______ Blood Pressure: ______ Temperature: ______ Other: ______
Snacks	Blood Sugar: ______ Blood Pressure: ______ Temperature: ______ Other: ______

- ☐ Fruit ☐ Vegetables ☐ Ginger Tea
- ☐ Grains & Cereals ☐ Fats

Daily Symptoms & Well-Being Tracker

DATE: ____ / ____ / ____

Today's Ratings

Pain	______ / 10	Anxiety	______ / 10	Went to bed	____ am / pm
Fatigue	______ / 10	Depression	______ / 10	Fell Asleep	____ am / pm
Weakness	______ / 10	Stress	______ / 10	Woke up	____ am / pm
Stiffness	______ / 10	Anger	______ / 10	Total Hours slept	________
General Mood	________			# of Disruptions	________

(Third column heading: **Sleep**)

Symptoms	Relief Attempts	Results Notes

Activity

- ☐ Walk - distance ________
- ☐ Physiotherapy
- ☐ Light Exercise
- ☐ Gym
- ☐ Housework
- ☐ ________
- ☐ ________

Medications taken

- ☐ Diabetes
- ☐ Blood Pressure
- ☐ Pain Management (Prescription)
- ☐ Pain (overcounter): ________
- ☐ Natural Therapies: ________
- ☐ Other: ________
- ☐ Other: ________

Medications

- ☐ No Change
- ☐ Dosage Changed
- ☐ from ________
- ☐ to ________
- ☐ Medication Changed
  - from ________
  - to ________

DAY

Daily Symptoms Tracker

Today,'s Dietary Intake

Drinks & Beverages

- ☐ Milk ☐ Juice ☐ Water
- ☐ Tea ☐ Coffee ☐ Soft / Energy Drink

Hydration

Breakfast	Blood Sugar: ____
____	Blood Pressure: ____
____	Temperature: ____
____	Other: ____
Lunch	
____	Blood Sugar: ____
____	Blood Pressure: ____
____	Temperature: ____
____	Other: ____
Dinner	
____	Blood Sugar: ____
____	Blood Pressure: ____
____	Temperature: ____
____	Other: ____
____	
Snacks	
____	Blood Sugar: ____
____	Blood Pressure: ____
____	Temperature: ____
____	Other: ____

- ☐ Fruit ☐ Vegetables ☐ Ginger Tea
- ☐ Grains & Cereals ☐ Fats

Daily Symptoms & Well-Being Tracker

DATE: ____ / ____ / ____

Today's Ratings

Pain	______ / 10	Anxiety	______ / 10	**Sleep**	
Fatigue	______ / 10	Depression	______ / 10	Went to bed	____ am / pm
Weakness	______ / 10	Stress	______ / 10	Fell Asleep	____ am / pm
Stiffness	______ / 10	Anger	______ / 10	Woke up	____ am / pm
General Mood	______			Total Hours slept	______
				# of Disruptions	______

Symptoms	Relief Attempts	Results Notes

Activity

- ☐ Walk - distance ______
- ☐ Physiotherapy
- ☐ Light Exercise
- ☐ Gym
- ☐ Housework
- ☐ ______
- ☐ ______

Medications taken

- ☐ Diabetes
- ☐ Blood Pressure
- ☐ Pain Management (Prescription)
- ☐ Pain (overcounter): ______
- ☐ Natural Therapies: ______
- ☐ Other: ______
- ☐ Other: ______

Medications

- ☐ No Change
- ☐ Dosage Changed
- ☐ from ______
- ☐ to ______
- ☐ Medication Changed
  - from ______
  - to ______

DAY

Today,'s Dietary Intake

Drinks & Beverages

- ☐ Milk ☐ Juice ☐ Water
- ☐ Tea ☐ Coffee ☐ Soft / Energy Drink

Hydration

Breakfast	
	Blood Sugar:
	Blood Pressure:
	Temperature:
	Other:

Lunch	
	Blood Sugar:
	Blood Pressure:
	Temperature:
	Other:

Dinner	
	Blood Sugar:
	Blood Pressure:
	Temperature:
	Other:

Snacks	
	Blood Sugar:
	Blood Pressure:
	Temperature:
	Other:

- ☐ Fruit ☐ Vegetables ☐ Ginger Tea
- ☐ Grains & Cereals ☐ Fats

Weekly Summary

	Monday	Tuesday	Wednesday	Thursday	Friday	Saturday	Sunday
Pain							
Fatigue							
Weakness							
Stiffness							
Sleep (total Hours)							
# Disruptions							

Instructions:

Use the dots and dashes below to graph your ratings for the week – it helps to see things visually.

The bottom -- equals 0; the middle -- equals 5; and the top ◆ equals 10

Weekly Summary

	Monday	Tuesday	Wednesday	Thursday	Friday	Saturday	Sunday
Anxiety							
Depression							
Stress							
Anger							
Brain Fog / Forgetfulness							

Daily Symptoms & Well-Being Tracker

DATE: ____ / ____ / ____

Today's Ratings

Pain ________ / 10
Fatigue ________ / 10
Weakness ________ / 10
Stiffness ________ / 10
General Mood ________

Anxiety ________ / 10
Depression ________ / 10
Stress ________ / 10
Anger ________ / 10

Sleep

Went to bed ____ am / pm
Fell Asleep ____ am / pm
Woke up ____ am / pm
Total Hours slept ________
# of Disruptions ________

Symptoms	Relief Attempts	Results Notes

Activity

- ☐ Walk - distance ________
- ☐ Physiotherapy
- ☐ Light Exercise
- ☐ Gym
- ☐ Housework
- ☐ ________
- ☐ ________

Medications taken

- ☐ Diabetes
- ☐ Blood Pressure
- ☐ Pain Management (Prescription)
- ☐ Pain (overcounter): ________
- ☐ Natural Therapies: ________
- ☐ Other: ________
- ☐ Other: ________

Medications

- ☐ No Change
- ☐ Dosage Changed
- ☐ from ________
- ☐ to ________
- ☐ Medication Changed
  - from ________
  - to ________

Today,'s Dietary Intake

DAY

Drinks & Beverages

- ☐ Milk
- ☐ Juice
- ☐ Water
- ☐ Tea
- ☐ Coffee
- ☐ Soft / Energy Drink

Hydration

Breakfast

Blood Sugar: ____

Blood Pressure: ____

Temperature: ____

Other: ____

Lunch

Blood Sugar: ____

Blood Pressure: ____

Temperature: ____

Other: ____

Dinner

Blood Sugar: ____

Blood Pressure: ____

Temperature: ____

Other: ____

Snacks

Blood Sugar: ____

Blood Pressure: ____

Temperature: ____

Other: ____

- ☐ Fruit
- ☐ Vegetables
- ☐ Ginger Tea
- ☐ Grains & Cereals
- ☐ Fats

Daily Symptoms & Well-Being Tracker

DATE: ____ / ____ / ____

Today's Ratings

Pain ________ / 10
Fatigue ________ / 10
Weakness ________ / 10
Stiffness ________ / 10
General Mood ____________

Anxiety ________ / 10
Depression ________ / 10
Stress ________ / 10
Anger ________ / 10

Sleep

Went to bed ____ am / pm
Fell Asleep ____ am / pm
Woke up ____ am / pm
Total Hours slept ____________
# of Disruptions ____________

Symptoms	Relief Attempts	Results Notes

Activity

- ☐ Walk - distance ________
- ☐ Physiotherapy
- ☐ Light Exercise
- ☐ Gym
- ☐ Housework
- ☐ ____________
- ☐ ____________

Medications taken

- ☐ Diabetes
- ☐ Blood Pressure
- ☐ Pain Management (Prescription)
- ☐ Pain (overcounter): ____________
- ☐ Natural Therapies: ____________
- ☐ Other: ____________
- ☐ Other: ____________

Medications

- ☐ No Change
- ☐ Dosage Changed
- ☐ from ____________
- ☐ to ____________
- ☐ Medication Changed

from ____________

to ____________

DAY

Today,'s Dietary Intake

Drinks & Beverages

- ☐ Milk ☐ Juice ☐ Water
- ☐ Tea ☐ Coffee ☐ Soft / Energy Drink

Hydration

Breakfast

Blood Sugar: ____
Blood Pressure: ____
Temperature: ____
Other: ____

Lunch

Blood Sugar: ____
Blood Pressure: ____
Temperature: ____
Other: ____

Dinner

Blood Sugar: ____
Blood Pressure: ____
Temperature: ____
Other: ____

Snacks

Blood Sugar: ____
Blood Pressure: ____
Temperature: ____
Other: ____

- ☐ Fruit ☐ Vegetables ☐ Ginger Tea
- ☐ Grains & Cereals ☐ Fats

Daily Symptoms & Well-Being Tracker

DATE: ____ / ____ / ____

Today's Ratings

Pain	______ / 10	Anxiety	______ / 10	Went to bed	____ am / pm
Fatigue	______ / 10	Depression	______ / 10	Fell Asleep	____ am / pm
Weakness	______ / 10	Stress	______ / 10	Woke up	____ am / pm
Stiffness	______ / 10	Anger	______ / 10	Total Hours slept	______
General Mood	______			# of Disruptions	______

Sleep

Symptoms	Relief Attempts	Results Notes

Activity

- ☐ Walk - distance ______
- ☐ Physiotherapy
- ☐ Light Exercise
- ☐ Gym
- ☐ Housework
- ☐ ______
- ☐ ______

Medications taken

- ☐ Diabetes
- ☐ Blood Pressure
- ☐ Pain Management (Prescription)
- ☐ Pain (overcounter): ______
- ☐ Natural Therapies: ______
- ☐ Other: ______
- ☐ Other: ______

Medications

- ☐ No Change
- ☐ Dosage Changed
- ☐ from ______
- ☐ to ______
- ☐ Medication Changed
  - from ______
  - to ______

DAY

Today,'s Dietary Intake

Drinks & Beverages

- ☐ Milk ☐ Juice ☐ Water
- ☐ Tea ☐ Coffee ☐ Soft / Energy Drink

Hydration

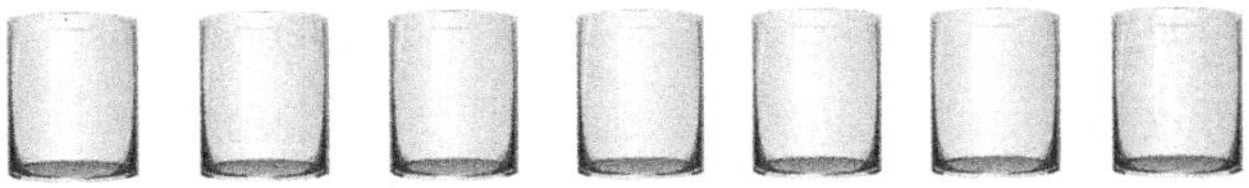

Breakfast

Blood Sugar: ____________
Blood Pressure: ____________
Temperature: ____________
Other: ____________

Lunch

Blood Sugar: ____________
Blood Pressure: ____________
Temperature: ____________
Other: ____________

Dinner

Blood Sugar: ____________
Blood Pressure: ____________
Temperature: ____________
Other: ____________

Snacks

Blood Sugar: ____________
Blood Pressure: ____________
Temperature: ____________
Other: ____________

- ☐ Fruit ☐ Vegetables ☐ Ginger Tea
- ☐ Grains & Cereals ☐ Fats

Daily Symptoms & Well-Being Tracker

DATE: ____ / ____ / ____

Today's Ratings

Pain ________ / 10

Fatigue ________ / 10

Weakness ________ / 10

Stiffness ________ / 10

General Mood ____________

Anxiety ________ / 10

Depression ________ / 10

Stress ________ / 10

Anger ________ / 10

Sleep

Went to bed _____ am / pm

Fell Asleep _____ am / pm

Woke up _____ am / pm

Total Hours slept ____________

# of Disruptions ____________

Symptoms	Relief Attempts	Results Notes

Activity

- ☐ Walk - distance ________
- ☐ Physiotherapy
- ☐ Light Exercise
- ☐ Gym
- ☐ Housework
- ☐ ____________
- ☐ ____________

Medications taken

- ☐ Diabetes
- ☐ Blood Pressure
- ☐ Pain Management (Prescription)
- ☐ Pain (overcounter): ____________
- ☐ Natural Therapies: ____________
- ☐ Other: ____________
- ☐ Other: ____________

Medications

- ☐ No Change
- ☐ Dosage Changed
- ☐ from ____________
- ☐ to ____________
- ☐ Medication Changed

from ____________

to ____________

DAY

Today,'s Dietary Intake

Drinks & Beverages

- ☐ Milk ☐ Juice ☐ Water
- ☐ Tea ☐ Coffee ☐ Soft / Energy Drink

Hydration

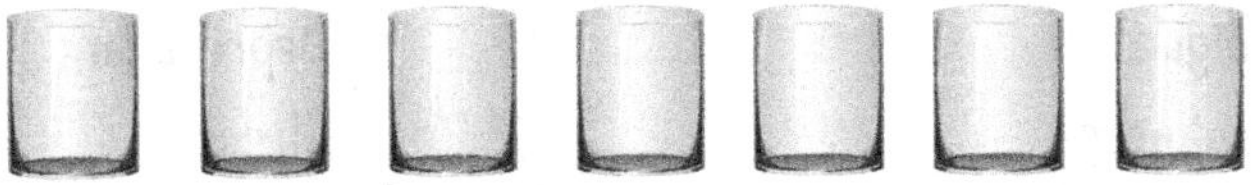

Breakfast

Blood Sugar: ____
Blood Pressure: ____
Temperature: ____
Other: ____

Lunch

Blood Sugar: ____
Blood Pressure: ____
Temperature: ____
Other: ____

Dinner

Blood Sugar: ____
Blood Pressure: ____
Temperature: ____
Other: ____

Snacks

Blood Sugar: ____
Blood Pressure: ____
Temperature: ____
Other: ____

- ☐ Fruit ☐ Vegetables ☐ Ginger Tea
- ☐ Grains & Cereals ☐ Fats

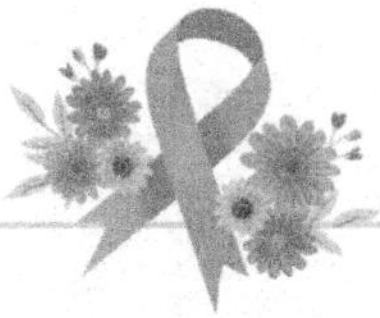

Daily Symptoms & Well-Being Tracker

DATE: ____ / ____ / ____

Today's Ratings

Pain	______ / 10	Anxiety	______ / 10
Fatigue	______ / 10	Depression	______ / 10
Weakness	______ / 10	Stress	______ / 10
Stiffness	______ / 10	Anger	______ / 10
General Mood	______		

Sleep

Went to bed	____ am / pm
Fell Asleep	____ am / pm
Woke up	____ am / pm
Total Hours slept	______
# of Disruptions	______

Symptoms	Relief Attempts	Results Notes

Activity

- ☐ Walk - distance ______
- ☐ Physiotherapy
- ☐ Light Exercise
- ☐ Gym
- ☐ Housework
- ☐ ______
- ☐ ______

Medications taken

- ☐ Diabetes
- ☐ Blood Pressure
- ☐ Pain Management (Prescription)
- ☐ Pain (overcounter): ______
- ☐ Natural Therapies: ______
- ☐ Other: ______
- ☐ Other: ______

Medications

- ☐ No Change
- ☐ Dosage Changed
- ☐ from ______
- ☐ to ______
- ☐ Medication Changed
  - from ______
  - to ______

Daily Symptoms Tracker

Today,'s Dietary Intake

DAY

Drinks & Beverages

- ☐ Milk ☐ Juice ☐ Water
- ☐ Tea ☐ Coffee ☐ Soft / Energy Drink

Hydration

Breakfast

Blood Sugar: ______
Blood Pressure: ______
Temperature: ______
Other: ______

Lunch

Blood Sugar: ______
Blood Pressure: ______
Temperature: ______
Other: ______

Dinner

Blood Sugar: ______
Blood Pressure: ______
Temperature: ______
Other: ______

Snacks

Blood Sugar: ______
Blood Pressure: ______
Temperature: ______
Other: ______

- ☐ Fruit ☐ Vegetables ☐ Ginger Tea
- ☐ Grains & Cereals ☐ Fats

Daily Symptoms & Well-Being Tracker

DATE: ____ / ____ / ____

Today's Ratings

Pain ________ / 10
Fatigue ________ / 10
Weakness ________ / 10
Stiffness ________ / 10
General Mood ________

Anxiety ________ / 10
Depression ________ / 10
Stress ________ / 10
Anger ________ / 10

Sleep

Went to bed ____ am / pm
Fell Asleep ____ am / pm
Woke up ____ am / pm
Total Hours slept ________
# of Disruptions ________

Symptoms	Relief Attempts	Results Notes

Activity

- ☐ Walk - distance ________
- ☐ Physiotherapy
- ☐ Light Exercise
- ☐ Gym
- ☐ Housework
- ☐ ________
- ☐ ________

Medications taken

- ☐ Diabetes
- ☐ Blood Pressure
- ☐ Pain Management (Prescription)
- ☐ Pain (overcounter): ________
- ☐ Natural Therapies: ________
- ☐ Other: ________
- ☐ Other: ________

Medications

- ☐ No Change
- ☐ Dosage Changed
- ☐ from ________
- ☐ to ________
- ☐ Medication Changed
  from ________
  to ________

DAY

Today,'s Dietary Intake

Drinks & Beverages

- ☐ Milk ☐ Juice ☐ Water
- ☐ Tea ☐ Coffee ☐ Soft / Energy Drink

Hydration

Meal	Measurements
Breakfast	Blood Sugar: ____ Blood Pressure: ____ Temperature: ____ Other: ____
Lunch	Blood Sugar: ____ Blood Pressure: ____ Temperature: ____ Other: ____
Dinner	Blood Sugar: ____ Blood Pressure: ____ Temperature: ____ Other: ____
Snacks	Blood Sugar: ____ Blood Pressure: ____ Temperature: ____ Other: ____

- ☐ Fruit ☐ Vegetables ☐ Ginger Tea
- ☐ Grains & Cereals ☐ Fats

Daily Symptoms & Well-Being Tracker

DATE: ____ / ____ / ____

Today's Ratings

Pain	______ / 10	Anxiety	______ / 10	Went to bed	____ am / pm
Fatigue	______ / 10	Depression	______ / 10	Fell Asleep	____ am / pm
Weakness	______ / 10	Stress	______ / 10	Woke up	____ am / pm
Stiffness	______ / 10	Anger	______ / 10	Total Hours slept	______
General Mood	______			# of Disruptions	______

(Sleep)

Symptoms	Relief Attempts	Results Notes

Activity

- ☐ Walk - distance ______
- ☐ Physiotherapy
- ☐ Light Exercise
- ☐ Gym
- ☐ Housework
- ☐ ______
- ☐ ______

Medications taken

- ☐ Diabetes
- ☐ Blood Pressure
- ☐ Pain Management (Prescription)
- ☐ Pain (overcounter): ______
- ☐ Natural Therapies: ______
- ☐ Other: ______
- ☐ Other: ______

Medications

- ☐ No Change
- ☐ Dosage Changed
- ☐ from ______
- ☐ to ______
- ☐ Medication Changed
  - from ______
  - to ______

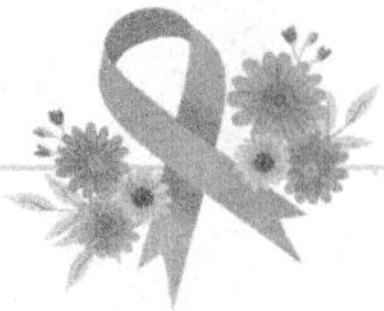

DAY

Today,'s Dietary Intake

Drinks & Beverages

☐ Milk ☐ Juice ☐ Water

☐ Tea ☐ Coffee ☐ Soft / Energy Drink

Hydration

Breakfast

Blood Sugar: ______

Blood Pressure: ______

Temperature: ______

Other: ______

Lunch

Blood Sugar: ______

Blood Pressure: ______

Temperature: ______

Other: ______

Dinner

Blood Sugar: ______

Blood Pressure: ______

Temperature: ______

Other: ______

Snacks

Blood Sugar: ______

Blood Pressure: ______

Temperature: ______

Other: ______

☐ Fruit ☐ Vegetables ☐ Ginger Tea

☐ Grains & Cereals ☐ Fats

Weekly Summary

	Monday	Tuesday	Wednesday	Thursday	Friday	Saturday	Sunday
Pain							
Fatigue							
Weakness							
Stiffness							
Sleep (total Hours)							
# Disruptions							

Instructions:

Use the dots and dashes below to graph your ratings for the week - it helps to see things visually.

The bottom -- equals 0; the middle -- equals 5; and the top ◆ equals 10

Weekly Summary

	Monday	Tuesday	Wednesday	Thursday	Friday	Saturday	Sunday
Anxiety							
Depression							
Stress							
Anger							
Brain Fog / Forgetfulness							

Daily Symptoms & Well-Being Tracker

DATE: ____ / ____ / ____

Today's Ratings

Pain	______ / 10	Anxiety	______ / 10	Went to bed	____ am / pm
Fatigue	______ / 10	Depression	______ / 10	Fell Asleep	____ am / pm
Weakness	______ / 10	Stress	______ / 10	Woke up	____ am / pm
Stiffness	______ / 10	Anger	______ / 10	Total Hours slept	______
General Mood	______			# of Disruptions	______

Symptoms	Relief Attempts	Results Notes

Activity

- ☐ Walk - distance ______
- ☐ Physiotherapy
- ☐ Light Exercise
- ☐ Gym
- ☐ Housework
- ☐ ______
- ☐ ______

Medications taken

- ☐ Diabetes
- ☐ Blood Pressure
- ☐ Pain Management (Prescription)
- ☐ Pain (overcounter): ______
- ☐ Natural Therapies: ______
- ☐ Other: ______
- ☐ Other: ______

Medications

- ☐ No Change
- ☐ Dosage Changed
- ☐ from ______
- ☐ to ______
- ☐ Medication Changed
- from ______
- to ______

Today,'s Dietary Intake

DAY

Drinks & Beverages

☐ Milk ☐ Juice ☐ Water

☐ Tea ☐ Coffee ☐ Soft / Energy Drink

Hydration

Breakfast

Blood Sugar: ______

Blood Pressure: ______

Temperature: ______

Other: ______

Lunch

Blood Sugar: ______

Blood Pressure: ______

Temperature: ______

Other: ______

Dinner

Blood Sugar: ______

Blood Pressure: ______

Temperature: ______

Other: ______

Snacks

Blood Sugar: ______

Blood Pressure: ______

Temperature: ______

Other: ______

☐ Fruit ☐ Vegetables ☐ Ginger Tea

☐ Grains & Cereals ☐ Fats

Daily Symptoms & Well-Being Tracker

DATE: ____ / ____ / ____

Today's Ratings

Pain	______ / 10	Anxiety	______ / 10
Fatigue	______ / 10	Depression	______ / 10
Weakness	______ / 10	Stress	______ / 10
Stiffness	______ / 10	Anger	______ / 10
General Mood	______		

Sleep

Went to bed	____ am / pm
Fell Asleep	____ am / pm
Woke up	____ am / pm
Total Hours slept	______
# of Disruptions	______

Symptoms	Relief Attempts	Results Notes

Activity

- ☐ Walk - distance ______
- ☐ Physiotherapy
- ☐ Light Exercise
- ☐ Gym
- ☐ Housework
- ☐ ______
- ☐ ______

Medications taken

- ☐ Diabetes
- ☐ Blood Pressure
- ☐ Pain Management (Prescription)
- ☐ Pain (overcounter): ______
- ☐ Natural Therapies: ______
- ☐ Other: ______
- ☐ Other: ______

Medications

- ☐ No Change
- ☐ Dosage Changed
- ☐ from ______
- ☐ to ______
- ☐ Medication Changed
  - from ______
  - to ______

Daily Symptoms Tracker

Today,'s Dietary Intake

DAY

Drinks & Beverages

- ☐ Milk ☐ Juice ☐ Water
- ☐ Tea ☐ Coffee ☐ Soft / Energy Drink

Hydration

Breakfast

Blood Sugar: ________
Blood Pressure: ________
Temperature: ________
Other: ________

Lunch

Blood Sugar: ________
Blood Pressure: ________
Temperature: ________
Other: ________

Dinner

Blood Sugar: ________
Blood Pressure: ________
Temperature: ________
Other: ________

Snacks

Blood Sugar: ________
Blood Pressure: ________
Temperature: ________
Other: ________

- ☐ Fruit ☐ Vegetables ☐ Ginger Tea
- ☐ Grains & Cereals ☐ Fats

Daily Symptoms & Well-Being Tracker

DATE: ____ / ____ / ____

Today's Ratings

Pain	______ / 10	Anxiety	______ / 10	Went to bed	____ am / pm
Fatigue	______ / 10	Depression	______ / 10	Fell Asleep	____ am / pm
Weakness	______ / 10	Stress	______ / 10	Woke up	____ am / pm
Stiffness	______ / 10	Anger	______ / 10	Total Hours slept	______
General Mood	______			# of Disruptions	______

Sleep

Symptoms	Relief Attempts	Results Notes

Activity

- ☐ Walk - distance ______
- ☐ Physiotherapy
- ☐ Light Exercise
- ☐ Gym
- ☐ Housework
- ☐ ______
- ☐ ______

Medications taken

- ☐ Diabetes
- ☐ Blood Pressure
- ☐ Pain Management (Prescription)
- ☐ Pain (overcounter): ______
- ☐ Natural Therapies: ______
- ☐ Other: ______
- ☐ Other: ______

Medications

- ☐ No Change
- ☐ Dosage Changed
- ☐ from ______
- ☐ to ______
- ☐ Medication Changed
  - from ______
  - to ______

Today,'s Dietary Intake

DAY

Drinks & Beverages

- ☐ Milk ☐ Juice ☐ Water
- ☐ Tea ☐ Coffee ☐ Soft / Energy Drink

Hydration

Breakfast

Blood Sugar: ______
Blood Pressure: ______
Temperature: ______
Other: ______

Lunch

Blood Sugar: ______
Blood Pressure: ______
Temperature: ______
Other: ______

Dinner

Blood Sugar: ______
Blood Pressure: ______
Temperature: ______
Other: ______

Snacks

Blood Sugar: ______
Blood Pressure: ______
Temperature: ______
Other: ______

- ☐ Fruit ☐ Vegetables ☐ Ginger Tea
- ☐ Grains & Cereals ☐ Fats

Daily Symptoms & Well-Being Tracker

DATE: ____ / ____ / ____

Today's Ratings

Pain	______ / 10	Anxiety	______ / 10		
Fatigue	______ / 10	Depression	______ / 10		
Weakness	______ / 10	Stress	______ / 10		
Stiffness	______ / 10	Anger	______ / 10		
General Mood	______				

Sleep

Went to bed	____ am / pm
Fell Asleep	____ am / pm
Woke up	____ am / pm
Total Hours slept	______
# of Disruptions	______

Symptoms	Relief Attempts	Results Notes

Activity

- ☐ Walk - distance ______
- ☐ Physiotherapy
- ☐ Light Exercise
- ☐ Gym
- ☐ Housework
- ☐ ______
- ☐ ______

Medications taken

- ☐ Diabetes
- ☐ Blood Pressure
- ☐ Pain Management (Prescription)
- ☐ Pain (overcounter): ______
- ☐ Natural Therapies: ______
- ☐ Other: ______
- ☐ Other: ______

Medications

- ☐ No Change
- ☐ Dosage Changed
- ☐ from ______
- ☐ to ______
- ☐ Medication Changed
- from ______
- to ______

DAY

Today.'s Dietary Intake

Drinks & Beverages

- ☐ Milk ☐ Juice ☐ Water
- ☐ Tea ☐ Coffee ☐ Soft / Energy Drink

Hydration

Breakfast	Blood Sugar: ____ Blood Pressure: ____ Temperature: ____ Other: ____
Lunch	Blood Sugar: ____ Blood Pressure: ____ Temperature: ____ Other: ____
Dinner	Blood Sugar: ____ Blood Pressure: ____ Temperature: ____ Other: ____
Snacks	Blood Sugar: ____ Blood Pressure: ____ Temperature: ____ Other: ____

- ☐ Fruit ☐ Vegetables ☐ Ginger Tea
- ☐ Grains & Cereals ☐ Fats

Daily Symptoms & Well-Being Tracker

DATE: ____ / ____ / ____

Today's Ratings

Pain ________ / 10
Fatigue ________ / 10
Weakness ________ / 10
Stiffness ________ / 10
General Mood ________

Anxiety ________ / 10
Depression ________ / 10
Stress ________ / 10
Anger ________ / 10

Sleep

Went to bed ____ am / pm
Fell Asleep ____ am / pm
Woke up ____ am / pm
Total Hours slept ________
# of Disruptions ________

Symptoms	Relief Attempts	Results Notes

Activity

- ☐ Walk - distance ________
- ☐ Physiotherapy
- ☐ Light Exercise
- ☐ Gym
- ☐ Housework
- ☐ ________
- ☐ ________

Medications taken

- ☐ Diabetes
- ☐ Blood Pressure
- ☐ Pain Management (Prescription)
- ☐ Pain (overcounter): ________
- ☐ Natural Therapies: ________
- ☐ Other: ________
- ☐ Other: ________

Medications

- ☐ No Change
- ☐ Dosage Changed
- ☐ from ________
- ☐ to ________
- ☐ Medication Changed
  - from ________
  - to ________

DAY

Today,'s Dietary Intake

Drinks & Beverages

- ☐ Milk ☐ Juice ☐ Water
- ☐ Tea ☐ Coffee ☐ Soft / Energy Drink

Hydration

☐ ☐ ☐ ☐ ☐ ☐ ☐

Breakfast	Blood Sugar:
	Blood Pressure:
	Temperature:
	Other:
Lunch	
	Blood Sugar:
	Blood Pressure:
	Temperature:
	Other:
Dinner	
	Blood Sugar:
	Blood Pressure:
	Temperature:
	Other:
Snacks	
	Blood Sugar:
	Blood Pressure:
	Temperature:
	Other:

- ☐ Fruit ☐ Vegetables ☐ Ginger Tea
- ☐ Grains & Cereals ☐ Fats

Daily Symptoms & Well-Being Tracker

DATE: ____ / ____ / ____

Today's Ratings

Pain	______ / 10	Anxiety	______ / 10		
Fatigue	______ / 10	Depression	______ / 10		
Weakness	______ / 10	Stress	______ / 10		
Stiffness	______ / 10	Anger	______ / 10		
General Mood	______				

Sleep

Went to bed	____ am / pm
Fell Asleep	____ am / pm
Woke up	____ am / pm
Total Hours slept	______
# of Disruptions	______

Symptoms	Relief Attempts	Results Notes

Activity

- ☐ Walk - distance ______
- ☐ Physiotherapy
- ☐ Light Exercise
- ☐ Gym
- ☐ Housework
- ☐ ______
- ☐ ______

Medications taken

- ☐ Diabetes
- ☐ Blood Pressure
- ☐ Pain Management (Prescription)
- ☐ Pain (overcounter): ______
- ☐ Natural Therapies: ______
- ☐ Other: ______
- ☐ Other: ______

Medications

- ☐ No Change
- ☐ Dosage Changed
- ☐ from ______
- ☐ to ______
- ☐ Medication Changed
- from ______
- to ______

Daily Symptoms Tracker

DAY

Today,'s Dietary Intake

Drinks & Beverages

- ☐ Milk ☐ Juice ☐ Water
- ☐ Tea ☐ Coffee ☐ Soft / Energy Drink

Hydration

Breakfast

Blood Sugar: ____
Blood Pressure: ____
Temperature: ____
Other: ____

Lunch

Blood Sugar: ____
Blood Pressure: ____
Temperature: ____
Other: ____

Dinner

Blood Sugar: ____
Blood Pressure: ____
Temperature: ____
Other: ____

Snacks

Blood Sugar: ____
Blood Pressure: ____
Temperature: ____
Other: ____

- ☐ Fruit ☐ Vegetables ☐ Ginger Tea
- ☐ Grains & Cereals ☐ Fats

Daily Symptoms & Well-Being Tracker

DATE: ____ / ____ / ____

Today's Ratings

Pain ________ / 10
Fatigue ________ / 10
Weakness ________ / 10
Stiffness ________ / 10
General Mood ________

Anxiety ________ / 10
Depression ________ / 10
Stress ________ / 10
Anger ________ / 10

Sleep

Went to bed ____ am / pm
Fell Asleep ____ am / pm
Woke up ____ am / pm
Total Hours slept ________
# of Disruptions ________

Symptoms	Relief Attempts	Results Notes

Activity

- ☐ Walk - distance ________
- ☐ Physiotherapy
- ☐ Light Exercise
- ☐ Gym
- ☐ Housework
- ☐ ________
- ☐ ________

Medications taken

- ☐ Diabetes
- ☐ Blood Pressure
- ☐ Pain Management (Prescription)
- ☐ Pain (overcounter): ________
- ☐ Natural Therapies: ________
- ☐ Other: ________
- ☐ Other: ________

Medications

- ☐ No Change
- ☐ Dosage Changed
- ☐ from ________
- ☐ to ________
- ☐ Medication Changed
  - from ________
  - to ________

DAY

Today,'s Dietary Intake

Drinks & Beverages

- ☐ Milk
- ☐ Juice
- ☐ Water
- ☐ Tea
- ☐ Coffee
- ☐ Soft / Energy Drink

Hydration

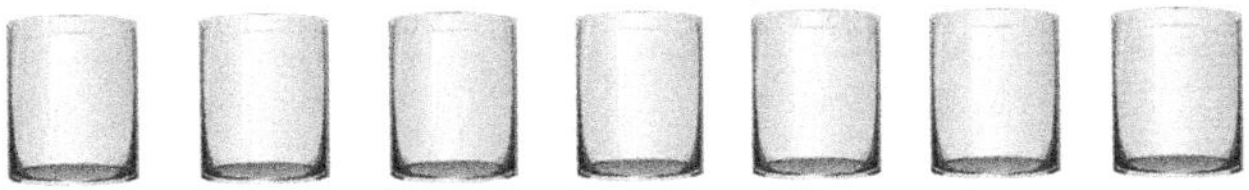

Breakfast

____

____

____

Blood Sugar: ________

Blood Pressure: ________

Temperature: ________

Other: ________

Lunch

____

____

____

____

Blood Sugar: ________

Blood Pressure: ________

Temperature: ________

Other: ________

Dinner

____

____

____

____

____

Blood Sugar: ________

Blood Pressure: ________

Temperature: ________

Other: ________

Snacks

____

____

____

____

Blood Sugar: ________

Blood Pressure: ________

Temperature: ________

Other: ________

- ☐ Fruit
- ☐ Vegetables
- ☐ Ginger Tea
- ☐ Grains & Cereals
- ☐ Fats

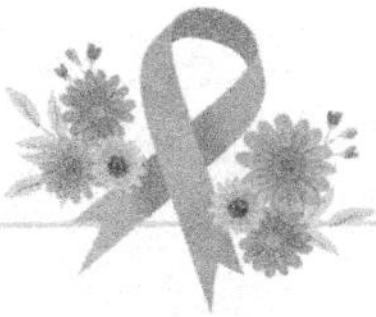

Weekly Summary

	Monday	Tuesday	Wednesday	Thursday	Friday	Saturday	Sunday
Pain							
Fatigue							
Weakness							
Stiffness							
Sleep (total Hours)							
# Disruptions							

Instructions:

Use the dots and dashes below to graph your ratings for the week - it helps to see things visually.

The bottom -- equals 0; the middle -- equals 5; and the top ◆ equals 10

Weekly Summary

	Monday	Tuesday	Wednesday	Thursday	Friday	Saturday	Sunday
Anxiety							
Depression							
Stress							
Anger							
Brain Fog / Forgetfulness							

Daily Symptoms & Well-Being Tracker

DATE: ____ / ____ / ____

Today's Ratings

Pain	____ / 10	Anxiety	____ / 10	Went to bed	____ am / pm
Fatigue	____ / 10	Depression	____ / 10	Fell Asleep	____ am / pm
Weakness	____ / 10	Stress	____ / 10	Woke up	____ am / pm
Stiffness	____ / 10	Anger	____ / 10	Total Hours slept	____
General Mood	____			# of Disruptions	____

Sleep

Symptoms	Relief Attempts	Results Notes

Activity

- ☐ Walk - distance ____
- ☐ Physiotherapy
- ☐ Light Exercise
- ☐ Gym
- ☐ Housework
- ☐ ____
- ☐ ____

Medications taken

- ☐ Diabetes
- ☐ Blood Pressure
- ☐ Pain Management (Prescription)
- ☐ Pain (overcounter): ____
- ☐ Natural Therapies: ____
- ☐ Other: ____
- ☐ Other: ____

Medications

- ☐ No Change
- ☐ Dosage Changed
- ☐ from ____
- ☐ to ____
- ☐ Medication Changed
  - from ____
  - to ____

DAY

Today,'s Dietary Intake

Drinks & Beverages

- ☐ Milk
- ☐ Juice
- ☐ Water
- ☐ Tea
- ☐ Coffee
- ☐ Soft / Energy Drink

Hydration

Breakfast

Blood Sugar: ______
Blood Pressure: ______
Temperature: ______
Other: ______

Lunch

Blood Sugar: ______
Blood Pressure: ______
Temperature: ______
Other: ______

Dinner

Blood Sugar: ______
Blood Pressure: ______
Temperature: ______
Other: ______

Snacks

Blood Sugar: ______
Blood Pressure: ______
Temperature: ______
Other: ______

- ☐ Fruit
- ☐ Vegetables
- ☐ Ginger Tea
- ☐ Grains & Cereals
- ☐ Fats

Daily Symptoms & Well-Being Tracker

DATE: ____ / ____ / ____

Today's Ratings

Pain	______ / 10	Anxiety	______ / 10	Went to bed	____ am / pm
Fatigue	______ / 10	Depression	______ / 10	Fell Asleep	____ am / pm
Weakness	______ / 10	Stress	______ / 10	Woke up	____ am / pm
Stiffness	______ / 10	Anger	______ / 10	Total Hours slept	______
General Mood	______			# of Disruptions	______

(Sleep)

Symptoms	Relief Attempts	Results Notes

Activity

- ☐ Walk - distance ______
- ☐ Physiotherapy
- ☐ Light Exercise
- ☐ Gym
- ☐ Housework
- ☐ ______
- ☐ ______

Medications taken

- ☐ Diabetes
- ☐ Blood Pressure
- ☐ Pain Management (Prescription)
- ☐ Pain (overcounter): ______
- ☐ Natural Therapies: ______
- ☐ Other: ______
- ☐ Other: ______

Medications

- ☐ No Change
- ☐ Dosage Changed
- ☐ from ______
- ☐ to ______
- ☐ Medication Changed
  - from ______
  - to ______

Today,'s Dietary Intake

DAY

Drinks & Beverages

- ☐ Milk
- ☐ Juice
- ☐ Water
- ☐ Tea
- ☐ Coffee
- ☐ Soft / Energy Drink

Hydration

Breakfast

Blood Sugar: ______
Blood Pressure: ______
Temperature: ______
Other: ______

Lunch

Blood Sugar: ______
Blood Pressure: ______
Temperature: ______
Other: ______

Dinner

Blood Sugar: ______
Blood Pressure: ______
Temperature: ______
Other: ______

Snacks

Blood Sugar: ______
Blood Pressure: ______
Temperature: ______
Other: ______

- ☐ Fruit
- ☐ Vegetables
- ☐ Ginger Tea
- ☐ Grains & Cereals
- ☐ Fats

Daily Symptoms & Well-Being Tracker

DATE: ____ / ____ / ____

Today's Ratings

Pain	______ / 10	Anxiety	______ / 10
Fatigue	______ / 10	Depression	______ / 10
Weakness	______ / 10	Stress	______ / 10
Stiffness	______ / 10	Anger	______ / 10
General Mood	______		

Sleep

Went to bed	____ am / pm
Fell Asleep	____ am / pm
Woke up	____ am / pm
Total Hours slept	______
# of Disruptions	______

Symptoms	Relief Attempts	Results Notes

Activity

- ☐ Walk - distance ______
- ☐ Physiotherapy
- ☐ Light Exercise
- ☐ Gym
- ☐ Housework
- ☐ ______
- ☐ ______

Medications taken

- ☐ Diabetes
- ☐ Blood Pressure
- ☐ Pain Management (Prescription)
- ☐ Pain (overcounter): ______
- ☐ Natural Therapies: ______
- ☐ Other: ______
- ☐ Other: ______

Medications

- ☐ No Change
- ☐ Dosage Changed
- ☐ from ______
- ☐ to ______
- ☐ Medication Changed
  - from ______
  - to ______

DAY

Today,'s Dietary Intake

Drinks & Beverages

- ☐ Milk ☐ Juice ☐ Water
- ☐ Tea ☐ Coffee ☐ Soft / Energy Drink

Hydration

☐ ☐ ☐ ☐ ☐ ☐ ☐

Breakfast

Blood Sugar: ______

Blood Pressure: ______

Temperature: ______

Other: ______

Lunch

Blood Sugar: ______

Blood Pressure: ______

Temperature: ______

Other: ______

Dinner

Blood Sugar: ______

Blood Pressure: ______

Temperature: ______

Other: ______

Snacks

Blood Sugar: ______

Blood Pressure: ______

Temperature: ______

Other: ______

- ☐ Fruit ☐ Vegetables ☐ Ginger Tea
- ☐ Grains & Cereals ☐ Fats

Daily Symptoms & Well-Being Tracker

DATE: ____ / ____ / ____

Today's Ratings

Pain	______ / 10	Anxiety	______ / 10		
Fatigue	______ / 10	Depression	______ / 10		
Weakness	______ / 10	Stress	______ / 10		
Stiffness	______ / 10	Anger	______ / 10		
General Mood	________				

Sleep

Went to bed	____ am / pm
Fell Asleep	____ am / pm
Woke up	____ am / pm
Total Hours slept	________
# of Disruptions	________

Symptoms	Relief Attempts	Results Notes

Activity

- ☐ Walk - distance ________
- ☐ Physiotherapy
- ☐ Light Exercise
- ☐ Gym
- ☐ Housework
- ☐ ________________
- ☐ ________________

Medications taken

- ☐ Diabetes
- ☐ Blood Pressure
- ☐ Pain Management (Prescription)
- ☐ Pain (overcounter): ________________
- ☐ Natural Therapies: ________________
- ☐ Other: ________________
- ☐ Other: ________________

Medications

- ☐ No Change
- ☐ Dosage Changed
- ☐ from ________________
- ☐ to ________________
- ☐ Medication Changed
  - from ________________
  - to ________________

Today,'s Dietary Intake

DAY

Drinks & Beverages

- ☐ Milk ☐ Juice ☐ Water
- ☐ Tea ☐ Coffee ☐ Soft / Energy Drink

Hydration

Breakfast

Blood Sugar: ____________
Blood Pressure: ____________
Temperature: ____________
Other: ____________

Lunch

Blood Sugar: ____________
Blood Pressure: ____________
Temperature: ____________
Other: ____________

Dinner

Blood Sugar: ____________
Blood Pressure: ____________
Temperature: ____________
Other: ____________

Snacks

Blood Sugar: ____________
Blood Pressure: ____________
Temperature: ____________
Other: ____________

- ☐ Fruit ☐ Vegetables ☐ Ginger Tea
- ☐ Grains & Cereals ☐ Fats

Daily Symptoms & Well-Being Tracker

DATE: ____ / ____ / ____

Today's Ratings

Pain	______ / 10	Anxiety	______ / 10	Went to bed	____ am / pm
Fatigue	______ / 10	Depression	______ / 10	Fell Asleep	____ am / pm
Weakness	______ / 10	Stress	______ / 10	Woke up	____ am / pm
Stiffness	______ / 10	Anger	______ / 10	Total Hours slept	______
General Mood	______			# of Disruptions	______

Symptoms	Relief Attempts	Results Notes

Activity

- ☐ Walk - distance ______
- ☐ Physiotherapy
- ☐ Light Exercise
- ☐ Gym
- ☐ Housework
- ☐ ______
- ☐ ______

Medications taken

- ☐ Diabetes
- ☐ Blood Pressure
- ☐ Pain Management (Prescription)
- ☐ Pain (overcounter): ______
- ☐ Natural Therapies: ______
- ☐ Other: ______
- ☐ Other: ______

Medications

- ☐ No Change
- ☐ Dosage Changed
- ☐ from ______
- ☐ to ______
- ☐ Medication Changed
  - from ______
  - to ______

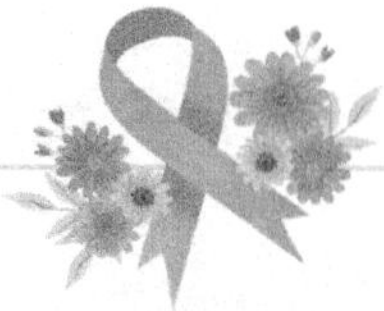

Today,'s Dietary Intake

DAY

Drinks & Beverages

- ☐ Milk ☐ Juice ☐ Water
- ☐ Tea ☐ Coffee ☐ Soft / Energy Drink

Hydration

Breakfast

Blood Sugar: ______
Blood Pressure: ______
Temperature: ______
Other: ______

Lunch

Blood Sugar: ______
Blood Pressure: ______
Temperature: ______
Other: ______

Dinner

Blood Sugar: ______
Blood Pressure: ______
Temperature: ______
Other: ______

Snacks

Blood Sugar: ______
Blood Pressure: ______
Temperature: ______
Other: ______

- ☐ Fruit ☐ Vegetables ☐ Ginger Tea
- ☐ Grains & Cereals ☐ Fats

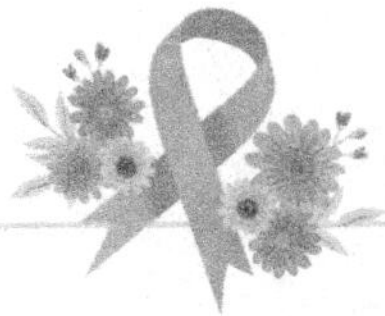

Daily Symptoms & Well-Being Tracker

DATE: ____ / ____ / ____

Today's Ratings

Pain	______ / 10	Anxiety	______ / 10		
Fatigue	______ / 10	Depression	______ / 10		
Weakness	______ / 10	Stress	______ / 10		
Stiffness	______ / 10	Anger	______ / 10		
General Mood	______				

Sleep

Went to bed	____ am / pm
Fell Asleep	____ am / pm
Woke up	____ am / pm
Total Hours slept	______
# of Disruptions	______

Symptoms	Relief Attempts	Results Notes

Activity

- ☐ Walk - distance ______
- ☐ Physiotherapy
- ☐ Light Exercise
- ☐ Gym
- ☐ Housework
- ☐ ______
- ☐ ______

Medications taken

- ☐ Diabetes
- ☐ Blood Pressure
- ☐ Pain Management (Prescription)
- ☐ Pain (overcounter): ______
- ☐ Natural Therapies: ______
- ☐ Other: ______
- ☐ Other: ______

Medications

- ☐ No Change
- ☐ Dosage Changed
- ☐ from ______
- ☐ to ______
- ☐ Medication Changed
  - from ______
  - to ______

DAY

Today,'s Dietary Intake

Drinks & Beverages

☐ Milk ☐ Juice ☐ Water

☐ Tea ☐ Coffee ☐ Soft / Energy Drink

Hydration

Breakfast

Blood Sugar: ______

Blood Pressure: ______

Temperature: ______

Other: ______

Lunch

Blood Sugar: ______

Blood Pressure: ______

Temperature: ______

Other: ______

Dinner

Blood Sugar: ______

Blood Pressure: ______

Temperature: ______

Other: ______

Snacks

Blood Sugar: ______

Blood Pressure: ______

Temperature: ______

Other: ______

☐ Fruit ☐ Vegetables ☐ Ginger Tea

☐ Grains & Cereals ☐ Fats

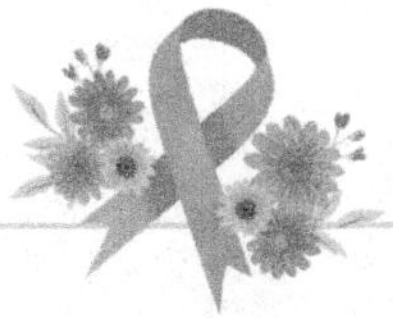

Daily Symptoms & Well-Being Tracker

DATE: ____ / ____ / ____

Today's Ratings

Pain	______	/ 10
Fatigue	______	/ 10
Weakness	______	/ 10
Stiffness	______	/ 10
General Mood	______	

Anxiety	______	/ 10
Depression	______	/ 10
Stress	______	/ 10
Anger	______	/ 10

Sleep

Went to bed	____	am / pm
Fell Asleep	____	am / pm
Woke up	____	am / pm
Total Hours slept	______	
# of Disruptions	______	

Symptoms	Relief Attempts	Results Notes

Activity

- ☐ Walk - distance ______
- ☐ Physiotherapy
- ☐ Light Exercise
- ☐ Gym
- ☐ Housework
- ☐ ______
- ☐ ______

Medications taken

- ☐ Diabetes
- ☐ Blood Pressure
- ☐ Pain Management (Prescription)
- ☐ Pain (overcounter): ______
- ☐ Natural Therapies: ______
- ☐ Other: ______
- ☐ Other: ______

Medications

- ☐ No Change
- ☐ Dosage Changed
- ☐ from ______
- ☐ to ______
- ☐ Medication Changed
  - from ______
  - to ______

DAY

Today,'s Dietary Intake

Drinks & Beverages

- ☐ Milk
- ☐ Juice
- ☐ Water
- ☐ Tea
- ☐ Coffee
- ☐ Soft / Energy Drink

Hydration

Breakfast

Blood Sugar: ______
Blood Pressure: ______
Temperature: ______
Other: ______

Lunch

Blood Sugar: ______
Blood Pressure: ______
Temperature: ______
Other: ______

Dinner

Blood Sugar: ______
Blood Pressure: ______
Temperature: ______
Other: ______

Snacks

Blood Sugar: ______
Blood Pressure: ______
Temperature: ______
Other: ______

- ☐ Fruit
- ☐ Vegetables
- ☐ Ginger Tea
- ☐ Grains & Cereals
- ☐ Fats

Weekly Summary

	Monday	Tuesday	Wednesday	Thursday	Friday	Saturday	Sunday
Pain							
Fatigue							
Weakness							
Stiffness							
Sleep (total Hours)							
# Disruptions							

Instructions:

Use the dots and dashes below to graph your ratings for the week - it helps to see things visually.

The bottom -- equals 0; the middle -- equals 5; and the top ◆ equals 10

Weekly Summary

	Monday	Tuesday	Wednesday	Thursday	Friday	Saturday	Sunday
Anxiety							
Depression							
Stress							
Anger							
Brain Fog / Forgetfulness							

My Notes

My Notes

My Notes

My Notes

My Notes

My Notes

Ginger Tea Recipe

Fresh ginger is commonly believed to reduce nausea, pain and inflammation.
A great way to add ginger to your diet is to make and drink Fresh Ginger Tea daily.

Ingredients

4 - 8 thin slices of fresh ginger
Hot (but not boiling) water
Sweetener (optional)

Method

* Finely slice fresh ginger and place in tea cup or coffee mug
* Heat Kettle - either switch off just before it boils, or boil kettle and wait 2 minutes
* Pour hot water over ginger slices
* Let steep for 2 to 3 minutes.
* Either spoon-out ginger slices and drink tea, or leave ginger slices in cup and drink
* You can reuse the sliced ginger to make 2 - 3 ginger teas.

Variations

* You can add other ingredients such as Lemon slices or tumeric powder to change up the flavour and increase the pain and inflammation reducting properties.

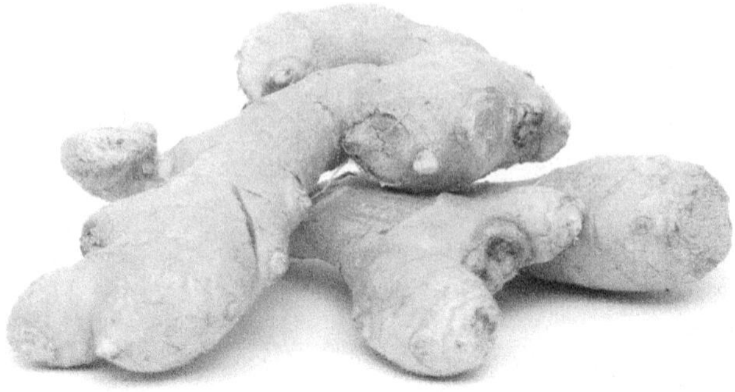

Made in the USA
Monee, IL
08 November 2026

67388664R00136